Fetal Monitoring in Practice

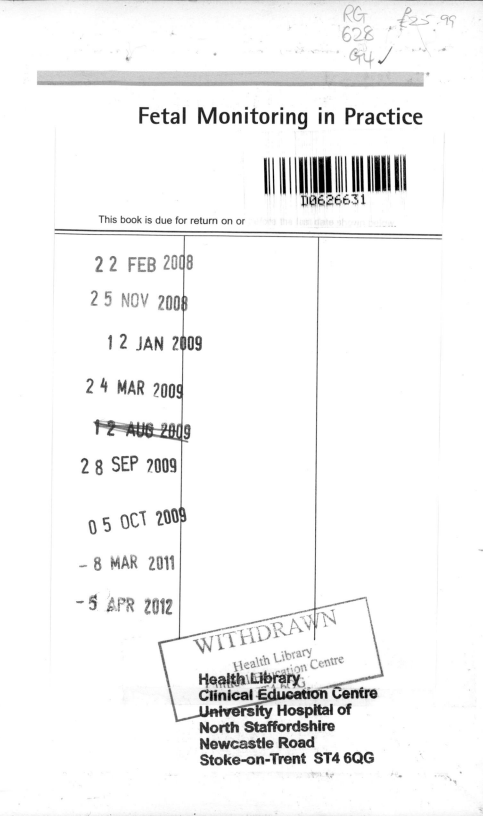

D0626631

This book is due for return on or before the last date shown below.

Dedicated to the health of mothers and babies

For Elsevier:

Commissioning Editor: Mairi McCubbin
Development Editor: Sheila Black
Project Manager: Gail Wright
Senior Designer: George Ajayi
Illustration Manager: Gillian Richards
Illustrator: Ian Ramsden

Fetal Monitoring in Practice

THIRD EDITION

Donald Gibb MD MRCP FRCOG MEWI

Independent Obstetrician and Gynaecologist, The Birth Company, London, UK

Formerly Director of Women's Services, Consultant Obstetrician and Gynaecologist, Honorary Senior Lecturer, King's College School of Medicine and Dentistry, King's College Hospital, London, UK

Sabaratnam Arulkumaran PhD FRCS(Ed) FRCOG

Professor and Head, Division of Obstetrics and Gynaecology, St George's University of London, UK

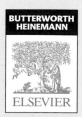

BUTTERWORTH
HEINEMANN

ELSEVIER

EDINBURGH LONDON NEW YORK OXFORD PHILADELPHIA ST LOUIS SYDNEY TORONTO 2008

BUTTERWORTH
HEINEMANN
ELSEVIER

BUTTERWORTH-HEINEMANN
An imprint of Elsevier Limited

First edition 1992
Second edition 1997

ISBN 978-0-443-10004-8

British Library Cataloguing in Publication Data
A catalogue record for this book is available from the British Library

Library of Congress Cataloging in Publication Data
A catalog record for this book is available from the Library of Congress

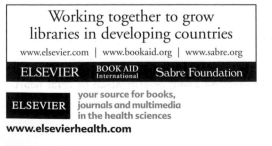

Working together to grow
libraries in developing countries

www.elsevier.com | www.bookaid.org | www.sabre.org

ELSEVIER   BOOK AID International   Sabre Foundation

ELSEVIER   your source for books,
journals and multimedia
in the health sciences
www.elsevierhealth.com

The publisher's policy is to use paper manufactured from sustainable forests

Printed in China

Contents

Preface

It is gratifying to have been asked to produce a third edition of this book. In 1992, with the first edition, we felt we were rather lone voices. Happily there have been developments in service provision, education and training that now complement our objectives. Litigation and complaint remain major issues, with the challenges that these bring. The messages remain the same. *The Fourth Confidential Enquiry into Stillbirths and Deaths in Infancy* (CESDI)[1] highlighted that 50% of intrapartum fetal deaths of those above 1500 gm with no chromosomal or congenital malformations could have been avoided. The main avoidable factors that were identified were inability to interpret CTG traces, failure to incorporate the clinical picture, delay in taking action and poor communication. We hope that the content of this book will at least partly contribute to resolving these issues.

In promoting safe motherhood as espoused by the World Health Organization, our objectives must be to optimize:

- the health of the mother
- the health of the offspring
- the emotional satisfaction of the mother and her family.

In developing countries with high maternal and perinatal mortality rates and limited resources, circumstances dictate that efforts are directed primarily at the first two objectives. In more-developed countries with less-frequent mortality and morbidity, attention can also be focused on the third goal.

The birth of a healthy baby is a universal aim. Although being born too early is the most common cause of perinatal loss, lack of oxygenation and nutrition is also a critical factor. Commonly referred to antenatally as intrauterine growth restriction and intrapartum as fetal distress, this condition presents a great challenge to obstetricians. However, in spite of technological developments in ultrasound and electronic fetal monitors, there has been some disillusion with the results of clinical application. Unexpectedly small babies are born with asphyxia, normal-size babies are born asphyxiated and normal-size babies are delivered operatively for 'fetal distress' in excellent condition. Those who believe in electronic fetal heart rate monitoring are often reminded by the sceptics that randomized controlled trials have failed to show any benefits of the procedure. There have been several controlled trials, some considering low-risk cases only and others taking high-risk and low-risk. Other trials have complemented electronic monitoring with pH measurement. Consistency of interpretation of the tracings agreed prospectively has not been a major feature of these studies. There is no consensus on how the procedure should be performed, the interpretation of results and the appropriate steps to be taken when the test is abnormal. Under these conditions the validity of such trials must be open to question. Of those studies, only the Dublin study[2] and that by Leveno et al[3] consisted of large enough numbers to reach meaningful conclusions. The Dublin study was performed on a selected population where only one-third of the intrapartum and neonatal deaths were included: preterm babies less than 29 weeks' gestation, cases with meconium-stained amniotic fluid, absent amniotic fluid and those who progressed rapidly in labour were excluded. Furthermore, only 80% allocated to the electronically monitored group were monitored and 11% had uninterpretable traces. Leveno et al[3] compared selective versus routine monitoring and showed no significant difference, except for a slightly higher caesarean section rate in routinely monitored cases. These studies highlight the need to identify the population to whom this technology should be applied. Intrapartum electronic fetal heart rate monitoring would not be expected to reduce a perinatal mortality rate because any effect would be swamped by deaths from other causes. Substantially less than one baby per 1000 births would be expected to die during labour under any circumstances. More subtle end-points need to be measured.

Technology in itself achieves nothing. It must be applied appropriately and correctly. Failure to understand this has resulted in the death of babies in spite of the intensive use of technology. Inappropriate application of technology and failure to take into account the clinical situation are common. The introduction of electronic fetal monitors has not been accompanied by any systematic attempt at education of the staff using them. The latter must be addressed and this is the prime objective of this book.

There is no such thing as 'no risk' in obstetrics. There is low risk and high risk, with a common phenomenon being a change in risk with time from the former to the latter; the converse does not occur. Excessive technology should not be applied to those who are manifestly at low risk. It may confer no benefit, can generate both non-medical and medical anxiety, and through subtle effects may cause significant harm. Women and their partners in developed societies sometimes seek natural childbirth (this really means birth with low technology and minimal intervention) and it is up to health service professionals to try to satisfy these needs. The unthinking application of technology is counterproductive. A relationship of trust and professionalism should bear fruit. It is acknowledged that the introduction of electronic fetal heart rate monitoring has contributed to an increase in the number of caesarean births. This is largely due to failure to understand the principles of the technique but may also be attributed to a fear of litigation. Both can be effectively countered.

We believe an extensive effort in education is required. We must approach new technologies after their benefit has been shown by proper randomized controlled trials. Most importantly, they should be introduced only with proper and continuing education. We should fully exploit the potential of fetal heart rate monitoring by education because all the new technology has fetal heart rate interpretation as the primary tool, the new technologies being adjuncts. We are in a position to contribute to this through extensive involvement in the labour wards. In the early 1980s we were privileged to be responsible for the deliveries under the care of the academic unit, Kandang Kerbau Hospital, Singapore. The total number of deliveries for the unit was 10 000 per year, with the government units supervising another 16 000 deliveries per year in the same labour ward. Epidural anaesthesia was not available; there was only one electronic fetal heart rate monitor and a considerable number of high-risk pregnancies. There were 28 beds in the high-risk delivery area and 18 beds in the low-risk delivery area. Ward rounds were no sooner finished than the next one started. More fetal monitors subsequently became available; however, there were never enough to monitor all of the mothers. Selection had to be undertaken and from this exercise we learned an enormous amount, through setting up clinical studies of selective electronic monitoring. The discipline of high-profile involvement in the labour wards has continued in the hospitals where we now work. Daily consultant ward rounds, caesarean section reviews, perinatal death reviews and joint discussions with the neonatologists all contribute to greater understanding. Confidence is required, in knowing as much when not to intervene as when to intervene. In a climate of possible complaint and litigation, inexperienced junior staff must be taught how to make these decisions. Confidence to encourage the low-risk mother in pursuit of natural childbirth to have appropriate minimal technology will come with this knowledge. Good communication between staff and with the mother is an excellent method of avoiding complaint and litigation.

Women in the labour ward are looked after by a team of midwives and doctors. There should be no demarcation of midwives' cases and doctors' cases. Low-risk mothers in normal labour will be looked after largely by midwives and this should be encouraged with the inclusion of phlebotomy, intravenous cannula siting and perineal suturing. Continuity of care will be enhanced and job satisfaction promoted. High-risk women will have a greater degree of medical input extending to the anaesthetist, neonatologist and senior obstetricians. Paradoxically, low-risk women pursuing natural birth should meet the medical staff sooner rather than later and be assured of the back-up position. The doctor may be seen as a fire prevention officer rather than a firefighter summoned in a moment of crisis. A team approach with respect for the contribution of each member will result in a healthy and productive working environment. Daily ward rounds and discussions form an important part of this approach. This does not involve taking a group of strangers to the bedside of a woman in labour; it involves meeting with the midwives, discussing each woman's situation and seeing those who need to be seen with the appropriate small group of immediate providers of care.

The government report, *Changing Childbirth*,[4] was an important challenge to the providers of care. It is not about power games between doctors and midwives but about a true team approach to woman-centred care. Midwives should have the responsibility of continuity of care for the low-risk mother. All, however, bear the responsibility for the safe passage of the baby. The midwives are in the front line as they deliver most of the bedside care in the labour ward. When the doctors become involved, it is important that the understanding and approach to fetal monitoring is consistent. It is artificial to divorce the education of the medical staff from that of the midwives. Midwives involved in caring for women in labour at home have a special responsibility. They require special skills in the application of clinical and low-technology monitoring.

The formation of the National Health Service Litigation Authority (NHSLA) with the associated Clinical Negligence Scheme for Trusts (CNST) in 1995, the Health Care Commission (HCC) and now the National Patient Safety Agency (NPSA), suggests a burgeoning of bureaucracy that requires much time and effort in paperwork. The work of these organizations is important in setting standards and regulation. We must be careful that investment in time and human resources to fulfil these obligations does not detract from patient care. These organizations have highlighted many matters that we know about that are relevant to our specialty.

The orientation of new or temporary staff must be undertaken. Thus all new staff in a labour ward should be provided with copies of the protocols and education in fetal monitoring, the Confidential Enquiry into Maternal and Child Health publication entitled *Why Mothers Die 2000–2002*,[5] and booklets from the Stillbirth and Neonatal Death Society, and other relevant documents should be freely available.

Case discussions and teaching sessions are very important. Circumspection and tact are important elements in review of cases with an adverse outcome. The aim is not to apportion blame but to learn from the experience and hopefully prevent a similar outcome in the future. Some of the examples in this book have been presented to us at seminars we have conducted. The participants, initially midwives but now including more doctors and legal professionals, have said that we have discussed things they already knew from experience but which they were not aware they knew. This has been very satisfying and is the true meaning of 'education'. We ourselves have learned a lot in a two-way process during such discussions.

We hope that those reading this book will be stimulated and will learn something to help them in promoting safer childbirth. They will above all realize that their task is easier and therefore more satisfying than they have been previously led to believe. It was the philosopher, Goethe, who said, 'It annoys man that the truth is so simple.'

London, 2008   *D. Gibb*
S. Arulkumaran

Acknowledgements

We are grateful to the following individuals and organizations for their contribution to earlier editions. The book would not have been possible without extensive collaboration. Doctors and midwives in King's College Hospital, London, and the National University Hospital, Singapore, were always interested in collecting and discussing traces. Staff attending seminars all over the world brought traces and provoked discussion.

Oxford Sonicaid, Huntleigh, Hewlett-Packard (Philips) and Corometrics (GE Health Care) supplied equipment on generous terms. The Wellcome Institute Library, London, gave permission for the reproduction of Figures 1.2 and 1.3.

Dr Jamal Zaidi collected traces. Mr Anthony Khoo in Singapore produced photographs. In London, Alex Dionysiou prepared artwork, with Yvonne Bartlett and Barry Pike producing photographs.

The staff at Elsevier provided encouragement and ongoing support.

Our families, Marie-Reine, Laurent and Pascale; Gayathri, Shankari, Nishkantha and Kailash, have tolerated our time-consuming obsession.

Thanks are expressed to all.

Chapter 1

Introduction

No written records of the detection of fetal life exist in western literature until the 17th century. Around 1650 Marsac, a French physician, was ridiculed in a poem by a colleague, Phillipe le Goust, for claiming to hear the heart of the fetus 'beating like the clapper of a mill'. It was not until 1818 that Francois-Isaac Mayor of Geneva, a physician, reported the fetal heart as audibly different from the maternal pulse heard by applying the ear directly to the pregnant mother's abdomen. Laennec, a physician working in Paris around 1816, was the father of the technique of auscultation of the adult heart and lungs. Le Jumeau, Vicomte de Kergaradec (Fig. 1.1), also a physician working with Laennec, became interested in applying this technique to other conditions including pregnancy. John Creery Ferguson, later to become first Professor of Medicine at the Queen's University of Belfast, visited Paris meeting Laennec and Le Jumeau. On his return to Dublin in 1827, Ferguson was the first person in the British Isles to describe the fetal heart sounds. He influenced Evory Kennedy, assistant master at the Rotunda Lying-in Hospital in Dublin, who wrote his famous work entitled *Observations on Obstetric Auscultation* in 1833. There was much argument over the technique of listening, some demanding the use of the stethoscope for reasons of decency only. At that time some doctors examined pregnant women through their clothing and this respect for the modesty of the woman must have inhibited the spread of obstetric auscultation. Anton Friedrich Hohl was the first to describe the design of the fetal stethoscope in 1834 (Fig. 1.2). Depaul modified this (Fig. 1.3) describing both in his *Traite D'Auscultation Obstetricale* in 1847. Although Pinard's name is most commonly associated with the stethoscope his version followed several others, only appearing in 1876. Many papers were subsequently published in a variety of languages elaborating the technique. In 1849 Kilian proposed the 'stethoscopical indications for forceps operation': 'The forceps must be applied under favourable conditions without delay when the fetal heart tones diminish to less

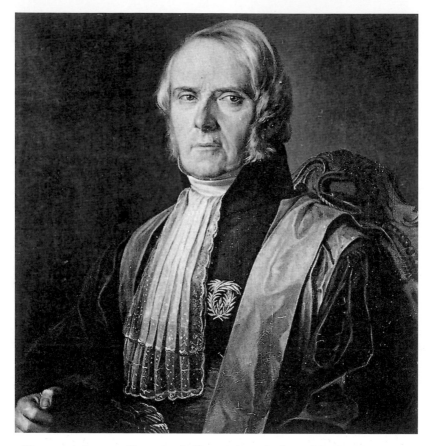

Figure 1.1 Jacques Alexandre de Kergaradec, robed as a Membre de l'Academie de Medicine Paris. (With thanks to Professor J.H.M. Pinkerton, Emeritus Professor of Midwifery and Gynaecology, Queen's University of Belfast)

than 100 beats per minute (bpm) or when they increase to 180 bpm or when they lose their purity of tone'. Winkel, in 1893, empirically set the limits of the normal heart rate at 120 bpm to 160 bpm. This has been carried forward for many years and reviewed in the light of the large amount of material produced by electronic recording.

If hearing the fetal heart was of any value then it was recognized that this was based on a very small sample of time subject to considerable observer variability. Listening for 15 seconds in 1 hour is only to sample 0.4% of the time. More continuous monitoring may be desirable. The advent of audiovisual techniques associated with the development of the film industry in the early 20th century set the

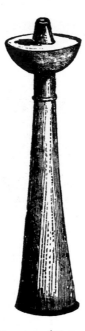

Figure 1.2 The Hohl fetal stethoscope (Wellcome Institute Library, London)

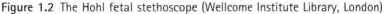

scene for technological developments that led to the equipment we have today. In 1953, while working in Lewisham Hospital, south-east London, Gunn and Wood reported 'The Amplification and Recording of Foetal Heart Sounds' in the *Proceedings of the Royal Society of Medicine*. In 1958, Hon pioneered electronic fetal monitoring in the USA. Caldeyro-Barcia in Uruguay and Hammacher in Germany reported their observations on the various heart rate patterns associated with so-called fetal distress. This set the scene for the production of the first commercially available fetal monitor by Hammacher and Hewlett-Packard in 1968 soon to be followed by Sonicaid in the UK. It is notable that Saling in Berlin had reported the use of fetal scalp blood sampling to study fetal pH two years prior to this in 1966. Fetal scalp blood pH assessment was developed in parallel with electronic monitoring, not as a sequel to it as might be assumed from our current practice.

The early equipment used phonocardiography, simply to listen and record sounds coming from the maternal abdomen as well as generating the fetal heart rate from the fetal electrocardiograph (ECG) from a fetal scalp electrode. Phonocardiography produces inferior traces because of the other extraneous sounds that confuse the picture. This problem was solved very quickly by the introduction of Doppler ultrasound transducers. When the Doppler transducer is applied to the maternal abdomen a Doppler signal is reflected from the moving

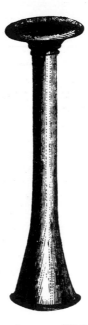

Figure 1.3 The Depaul fetal stethoscope (Wellcome Institute Library, London)

fetal heart, the location of which has already been determined by auscultation. The signal is altered by a moving structure according to the Doppler shift principle and received by the transducer in its altered form. The moving structure is usually the moving heart and the blood flowing through it. Ultrasound Doppler technology has improved considerably in recent years and the latest generation of monitors produce excellent quality external traces, comparable to those generated by direct ECG. The previous justification that rupture of the membranes and application of a fetal electrode are necessary in order to generate a good quality trace is no longer valid. This improvement can be largely attributed to the technique of autocorrelation or dual autocorrelation and the use of wide beams. Monitoring of both twins externally has presented problems because of interference between the two Doppler beams. That has been solved in the latest equipment by the use of two different frequencies, or the same frequency but distinguished by position using ultrasound 'windows' in the two ultrasound transducers so that the beams do not interfere with each other. The direct fetal ECG can be obtained by an external or internal technique. The external technique is only used in a research situation because the signal has to be electronically cleaned to remove the maternal ECG and electrical activity from the anterior abdominal wall. Direct detection of the fetal heart rate from a fetal electrode applied to the fetus at vaginal examination is used in clinical practice. This is commonly called a scalp electrode but is better termed a fetal electrode in view of its possible application to the breech. All machines provide an external tocography facility through a relatively simple strain gauge transducer. It should be appreciated that this provides only an indirect assessment of the uterine contractions. It indicates the frequency and duration of contractions but little about actual pressure or basal tone. In the unusual situation of requiring direct data about the intrauterine pressure, an intrauterine catheter is necessary with the relevant option in the machine. However, the climate of childbirth has retreated from the excessive use of invasive technology and the role of internal monitoring has become much more limited.

The clinical needs should be assessed and the specification of the machine required determined accordingly. A monitor to be used for antenatal monitoring does not require the intrapartum options and is therefore less expensive. Most modern monitors have similar specifications. The specification of a top-of-the-range intrapartum monitor is shown in Box 1.1.

Box 1.1 Specification of intrapartum monitor

Reliable
User friendly with operating manual and video
Robust with customized trolley

Fetal heart rate by external Doppler ultrasound (US) with
    autocorrelation
Fetal heart rate by fetal electrode (ECG)
Twin monitoring US and ECG
Twin monitoring US and US

Maternal heart rate
Event marker

External tocography
Internal tocography as an option

Mode, date and time printout
Keypad as an option

Automatic blood pressure, pulse and SaO_2 facility (an option
    selectively for high risk labours)

Antepartum monitors have become smaller. New models of hand-held Doptones include a digital display of the heart rate. Some models are waterproof for use in the water-labour scenario. Low-cost printers which can be attached to such devices are being developed. Such systems offer exciting possibilities to countries that have not yet started on the troublesome journey of extensive electronic fetal monitoring. They must be helped to avoid the costly mistakes made by the more developed countries. Technology should be appropriate, low cost and high quality.

The value of telemetry and telephone transmission of the fetal heart rate remains to be proven: investment should not be made in these options without a clear purpose. Telemetric transmission of the cardiotocograph (CTG) has become more practicable with improved technology in recent years, allowing the woman to remain mobile in early labour. However, more selective use of the technology has meant that some of the women who had telemetric monitoring do not actually require continuous electronic monitoring. The advent of mobile epidural anaesthesia and the use of water pools may rekindle interest in this kind of technology.

A solid trolley is an important investment to protect the machine during its busy life in the clinical area. Servicing, back-up and supplies of paper and electrodes must be assured. Modern machines have been factory tested to ensure proper functioning in any climate in the world. They are designed to be used 24 hours a day, 7 days a week. Although the concept of rest and recovery is valid for human beings, it is not necessary for such machines!

The twin option requires both transducers to be plugged in at the same time. In a monitor that prints two channels, one for each fetus, after monitoring twins one should be unplugged or there will be an empty channel on the paper creating a changed impression of scale and altered appreciation of the trace pattern. The electronic clock timings are battery dependent and require adjustment with time changes in the autumn and spring. CTG timings are important in record keeping.

An important step is to identify the midwifery and technical staff who will be responsible for day-to-day supervision and maintenance of this equipment. It is uncommon for such equipment to develop technical faults and defects will more often be user related. Simple housekeeping and in-service education will pay dividends. Not putting jelly on the tocograph transducer, not breaking the plugs by using push–pull rather than screw action, being careful that transducer cables are not run over and broken by trolley wheels and ensuring the use of the correct paper the right way round are fairly simple instructions sometimes not given due attention. An expensive piece of equipment requires common-sense care. It is a pity if equipment is out of action because of user errors.

Chapter 2

Clinical assessment and recording

The process of birth is a hazardous journey for any individual. The complete journey is from conception until discharge from hospital of the healthy mother and baby. The continuum of fetal health involves antenatal wellbeing and neonatal wellbeing. This is the modern concept of perinatology. As few, if any, obstetricians are also neonatologists a clearer concept is maternofetal medicine. Although we are not neonatologists, we must maintain an interest in our in-utero patient during his or her stay in the neonatal unit, just as the neonatologist will have joined us in assessment and counselling of the high-risk mother antenatally.

The part of the journey with which we are particularly concerned is that of labour and birth. The concept of preparation is an important one and for our purposes we consider this journey to start with admission to the labour ward. When we prepare for a journey we ensure that we are in good health, our vehicle is in good condition, the roads we will drive on are safe and that we have a good insurance policy. Admission to the labour ward is the time for such a review of the pregnant mother. Intrapartum events are a continuum of antenatal events. Many babies who get into difficulty in labour have already become compromised in the antenatal period and our surveillance system must be designed to find these fetuses and ensure their safe delivery. Assessment on admission helps us to look carefully for high risk factors previously undetected or new factors that have since appeared.

On admission to the labour ward the history is summarized taking particular note of high-risk factors such as previous perinatal loss, previous or existing intrauterine growth restriction, bleeding in pregnancy, diabetes mellitus, reduced fetal movements and a variety of other markers. Breech presentation and multiple pregnancies are obvious high-risk factors. On examination general features such as height, weight, blood pressure, temperature and signs of anaemia are reviewed. Before proceeding to vaginal examination, abdominal examination must be complete. This includes a measurement of abdominal size, an estimate of fetal size, lie, presentation and station of the presenting part. The nature of the contractions, amniotic fluid volume estimation and auscultation of the fetal heart complete this procedure. Traditionally the size of the abdomen and fetus is assessed subjectively. The value of formalizing this with an objective value has been suggested in recent years.[6] A measure of the fundosymphysis height (FSH) in centimetres (Figs 2.1 and 2.2) provides a reliable guide to fetal size so long as the observers have been trained in the technique.[7,8] The fundus should not be actively pushed down during

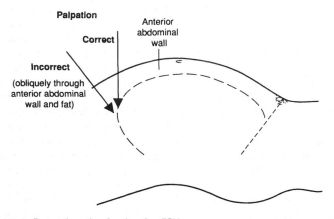

Figure 2.1 Detecting the fundus for FSH measurement

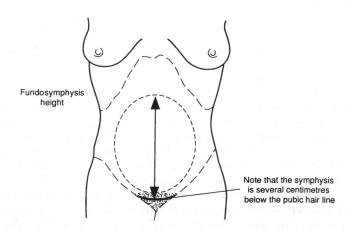

Figure 2.2 Measurement of FSH

the palpation, and the height from the top of the fundus (without correcting the uterus to the midline) to the upper margin of the symphysis pubis should be measured. Ideally a blinded measurement using the blank side of a tape measure is desirable. Due attention should be paid to the possible confounding factors of obesity, polyhydramnios, fibroids or unusual physical characteristics of the mother. After 20 weeks' gestation the FSH should be equivalent to the gestational age in centimetres ±2 cm up to 36 weeks, and ±3 cm after 36 weeks. No test should be subjected to unrealistic expectations. A tape measure is cheap, available and reasonably reliable with little inter- or intraobserver variation.[9] We are not good at identifying small babies in utero; this is obvious from studies of adverse perinatal outcome. The reduced fundosymphysis height may indicate a small fetus who may be suffering from chronic asphyxia (intrauterine growth restriction; see Ch. 6). Such a fetus is more likely to develop an abnormal heart rate pattern before, and particularly in, labour. A suspicion of a large fetus is also important so that we can anticipate and prepare for mechanical problems. A history of big babies, shoulder dystocia and diabetes mellitus are all important indicators. A rewarding exercise is recording the estimated fetal weight on the partogram. With experience and regular practice this becomes reliable. Management may be altered if abnormal labour progress becomes manifest and there is a likelihood of cephalopelvic disproportion. Marking 'Beware shoulder dystocia' in the 'special features' box on the partogram of women carrying large babies, and especially with a history of shoulder dystocia, is an important preventative measure. Medical help will be organized to be readily available in the second stage of labour.

Abdominal examination is performed before vaginal examination.

Vaginal examination is undertaken after abdominal palpation. Progressive changes in the uterine cervix permit a diagnosis of labour to be made in the presence of painful uterine contractions occurring at least once every 10 min with or without a show or spontaneous rupture of the membranes. This is an important diagnosis. Without it the mother will not be kept in the labour ward with the likelihood of ill-advised intervention. In this situation the best decision is often to do nothing rather than to do something. Inexperienced medical staff sometimes seem to feel an irrational pressure to intervene. Antenatal education should include an objective of the mother not admitting herself to hospital too early in labour. Some hospitals send a midwife to perform an assessment at home. At this stage the contractions are likely to be at least one in every 5 min and quite painful. If there has been spontaneous rupture of the membranes without labour being present (prelabour rupture of the membranes) then digital examination should not be performed unless a decision has already

mother who, on history and examination, is low risk assures a healthy fetus for the next 4 hours unless one of four events supervenes:

1. placental abruption
2. umbilical cord prolapse
3. injudicious use of oxytocics
4. imprudent application of instruments.

Placental abruption is characterized by pain, anxiety, tachycardia and often bleeding; a good midwife or doctor should suspect and detect it. It is estimated that 1 in 5 may have minimal or no symptoms and the condition diagnosed retrospectively.[10] Umbilical cord prolapse occurs after rupture of the membranes with a high presenting part. Good midwifery and medical practice should detect this early when it occurs in the labour ward and the outcome for this condition is excellent when properly treated. The proper use of oxytocics and appropriate electronic monitoring (see Ch. 10) and the proper use of instruments are promoted by education and training. Death of a normally-formed term fetus within 4 hours of a normal CTG is a rare event but certainly can occur with a serious placental abruption for which there may be no warning sign. A fetus can die of placental abruption within 15 min of a normal CTG.

The importance of clinical sense cannot be overemphasized. Figure 2.4 shows the 'complete' CTG machine including an accompanying tape measure and fetal stethoscope. Why the fetal stethoscope? The CTG shown in Figure 2.5 was undertaken in a mother admitted

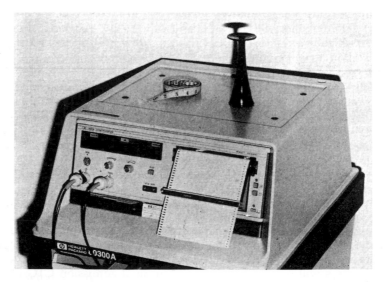

Figure 2.4 'Complete' fetal monitor

complaining of reduced fetal movements. The fetal stethoscope was not used and the ultrasound transducer was applied directly to the maternal abdomen. The mother was reassured that the baby was healthy; however a macerated stillbirth occurred 1 hour later. The heart rate picked up was the maternal pulse from a major vessel with the ultrasound beam having passed through the dead fetus. The mother had a tachycardia on account of her anxiety. Figure 2.6 is the trace obtained when the mother was admitted draining thick meconium and a scalp electrode was applied with some urgency. The

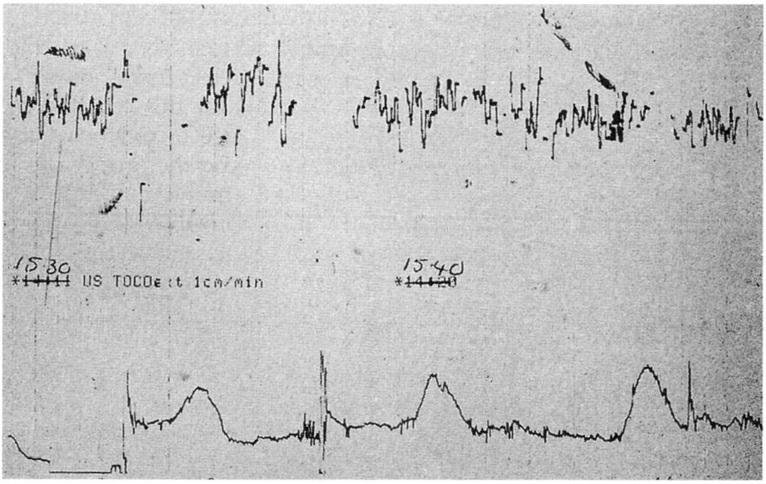

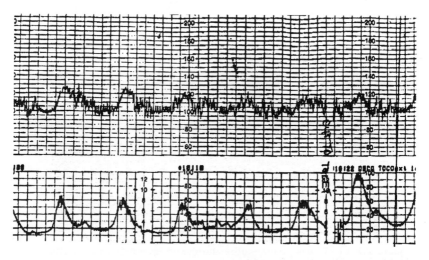

Figure 2.5 CTG of dead baby – ultrasound

Figure 2.6 CTG of dead baby – fetal electrode

midwives were reassured by the trace but the baby was born shortly thereafter as a macerated stillbirth. It was growth restricted and had died of hypoxia some time before. On account of oligohydramnios the fetal buttocks were in contact with the fundus which in turn was in contact with the diaphragm and the path of transmission of the maternal electrocardiograph (ECG) through the fetus is clear. The scalp electrode may therefore capture the maternal ECG when the fetus is dead. The stethoscope must always be used to establish a fetal pulse different from the maternal pulse.

Figure 2.7 is the trace obtained when another mother attended, not in labour but complaining of reduced fetal movements. The midwives applied the Hewlett-Packard 1350 fetal monitor which includes a fetal movement detector in the ultrasound transducer. The black lines in the middle of the trace indicate movements. The mother returned some hours later and delivered a macerated stillbirth. The ultrasound had again picked up the mother's pulse but, more worryingly, the movements detected were not fetal movements but maternal intestinal activity or other maternal movement. It should be noted that adult heart rate recordings also show baseline variability and accelerations. Prolonged accelerations at the time of uterine contractions and increased variability are characteristic of the maternal heart rate in the second stage when the mother has uterine contractions and she is bearing down.[11] An increasingly recognized mistake occurs when the monitor records the maternal heart rate with accelerations (Fig. 2.8) instead of the FHR with decelerations that should be seen with head compression. This may obscure a trace that would be showing a prolonged deceleration requiring delivery. Proper clinical application and relating the FHR patterns carefully to contractions should help us to avoid these tragic pitfalls. The mother's pulse rate

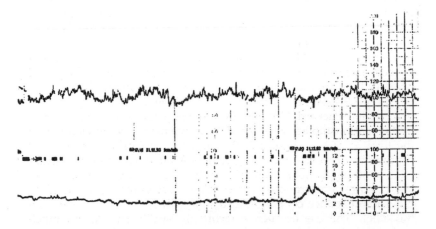

Figure 2.7 CTG of dead baby – ultrasound with fetal movement profile

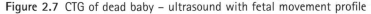

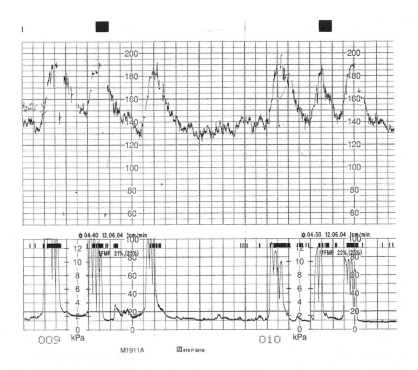

Figure 2.8 Recording in the second stage of labour – the monitor is recording the maternal heart rate which is increasing with uterine contractions and bearing-down efforts with increased baseline variability, instead of exhibiting the typical head compression FHR decelerations

should be correlated to the FHR and annotated at the beginning of the trace. The Medical Devices Agency in the UK advise the fetal heart should be auscultated prior to the monitor being used, because the maternal heart rate may be detected. The maternal heart rate may be the same as the FHR or it may be doubled and at times increased by 50% based on the number of maternal pulses picked up and whether they are picked up continuously or intermittently.

Figure 2.9 shows the correct use of the 'kineto cardiotocograph' on the Hewlett-Packard 1350 monitor showing the physiological truth of the relationship between true fetal movements and acceleration of the fetal heart rate. Figure 2.10 shows the correct use of maternal continuous heart rate recording as now available on all intrapartum fetal monitors, demonstrating clearly that, not surprisingly, the adult heart shows accelerations and baseline variability. Understanding this should reduce confusion in distinguishing one heart rate from the other. The use of such a facility is ideally suited, but much underused, in the scenario of managing preterm labour with beta

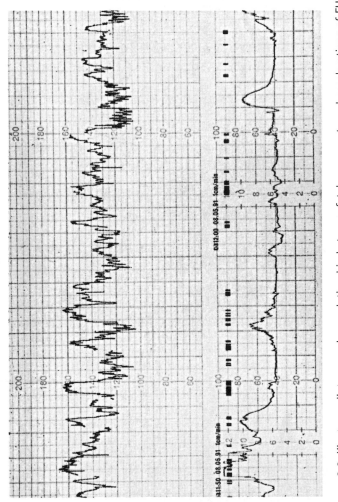

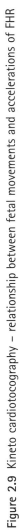

Figure 2.9 Kineto cardiotocography – relationship between fetal movements and accelerations of FHR

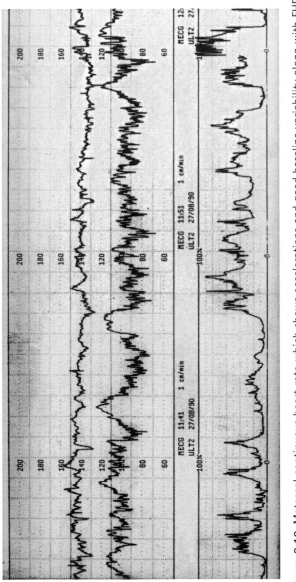
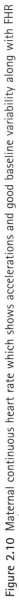

Figure 2.10 Maternal continuous heart rate which shows accelerations and good baseline variability along with FHR

sympathomimetic therapy. This issue of maternal tachycardia may be less of a problem with the use of atosiban.

The importance of clinical sense cannot be overemphasized.

Incidentally, Figure 2.5 also shows a common day-to-day error: the incorrect setting of the clock mechanism recording the time on the trace. This may be user error, particularly frequent after a seasonal time change, or the batteries in the machine may be running low. It should be very simply corrected.

Good communication with the mother and her partner is vital. Obstetric cases are unique in that they are not sick, as are patients in all other departments of the hospital. On the contrary, they are experiencing one of the most important events in their lives with enormous emotional impact. The intimacy of this should not be compromised except in the 'genuine interest' of safety for mother and child. This book should help us to recognize this genuine interest. Without this we will not earn the approbation of those who have entrusted their care to us.

Chapter 3

Electronic fetal monitoring: terminology

Even when we all speak one language there remain difficulties in communication because of differing use of terminology. This may be resolved by better understanding and consideration of terms and definitions agreed by the International Federation of Obstetrics and Gynaecology (FIGO) Subcommittee on Standards in Perinatal Medicine. These recommendations were published in 1987 in the *International Journal of Gynecology and Obstetrics*.[12] Recently the National Institute for Clinical Excellence (NICE) has published guidelines on fetal monitoring and they are largely used in this text.[13] Without a consistency of terminology we cannot have a consistency of interpretation.

Monitoring is first of all clinical and then complemented by technological methods. No cardiotocograph (CTG) can be interpreted without careful appraisal of the clinical situation. The following list illustrates particularly high-risk factors: prematurity, postmaturity, poor fetal growth, reduced fetal movements, meconium-stained amniotic fluid, bleeding in pregnancy, high blood pressure, breech presentation, multiple pregnancy and diabetes mellitus. This list could be extended indefinitely and yet would still only account for a minority of women delivering babies in most labour wards. Recognition of these factors is critical.

In the UK we refer to antepartum CTGs and intrapartum CTGs. In the USA antepartum CTGs are referred to as non-stress tests (NSTs). These are therefore distinguished from contraction stress tests (CSTs) where the contractions are stimulated by exogenous oxytocin. In the UK, CSTs are not performed and reliance is placed on other biophysical tests of fetal wellbeing. The admission test (CTG) is a natural contraction stress test using the contractions of early labour.

A fetal heart rate tracing should be technically adequate to warrant analysis. The pen heat should not be too high because it can produce a very dark trace, occasionally burning the paper, or too low, producing a faint trace. This can be adjusted on most machines; however, it is also affected by using the incorrect paper for the machine. The length of the CTG strip depends on the paper speed. In the UK it is usually 1 cm/min while in the USA it is 3 cm/min. As the pattern of the trace is dramatically altered by a change in paper speed this can lead to confusion. It should, therefore, be standardized. Because there is not much to be gained by the faster paper speed with a consequent greater consumption of paper the slower speed of 1 cm/min should be selected. Each vertical division on the paper is 1 cm and therefore 1 min. A tracing should be annotated fully. At the beginning of the trace the mother's name, reference number and pulse rate should be recorded. Modern machines automatically annotate the time and date; however, a human being has to ensure that they are correctly set in the software and changed as the clock time changes, notably with the onset of 'summer time'. The newest monitors have keypads or bar-code readers with which any other information may be recorded on the trace. It is important to relate vaginal examination, change of posture, epidural and other transient events to the fetal heart rate pattern, which could have medico-legal implications at a later date. The vertical scale on the paper should be standardized to display between 50 and 210 beats per min (bpm) in order for visual perception and interpretation to be consistent.

A tracing should be annotated fully.

The *baseline fetal heart rate* is the mean level of the fetal heart rate when this is stable, with accelerations and decelerations excluded. It is determined over a time period of 5 or 10 min and expressed in bpm. The rate may gradually change over time, however, for one particular period normally remains fairly constant. NICE has defined the normal range of the baseline fetal heart rate at term as 110–160 bpm.[13]

Rates between 100 and 110 bpm are classified as baseline *bradycardia* and as a suspicious feature. There is little concern if it is an uncomplicated baseline bradycardia defined as a trace that has accelerations, normal baseline variability and there are no decelerations. Close involvement in the labour ward shows us that this is a relatively frequent finding and the outcome is excellent (Fig. 3.1). Hypoxia should be suspected if the rate is below 100 bpm.

A range between 160 and 180 bpm is called a baseline *tachycardia* and is considered a suspicious feature. The outcome is good if it is an uncomplicated baseline tachycardia with accelerations, normal baseline variability and no decelerations. However, fetuses at term with a baseline heart rate of between 160 and 180 bpm should be carefully evaluated (Fig. 3.2a). A baseline rate of 150 bpm may fall within the normal range but is of major concern if the fetus had a heart rate of 120 bpm at the beginning of labour. Such a situation occurs in the late first stage and second stage of a prolonged labour

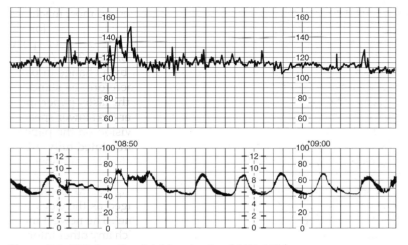

Figure 3.1 CTG: baseline fetal heart rate of 105–110 bpm

when the mother is tired, dehydrated and ketotic. If corrective measures are not undertaken the rate will rise to 160–170 bpm (Fig. 3.2b). This represents progressive asphyxia and is not an ideal scenario for a difficult instrumental vaginal delivery. Asphyxia is more likely to develop with a baseline rate of 160 compared to 110 bpm. This statement must be qualified before 34 weeks' gestation when the baseline fetal heart rate tends to be higher and a rate of up to 160 bpm is acceptable, provided accelerations are present and baseline variability is normal. Difficulties with identifying the baseline are considered in Chapter 5.

An *acceleration* is defined as a transient increase in heart rate of 15 bpm or more and lasting 15 s or more. The recording of at least two accelerations in a 20-min period is considered a reactive trace. Accelerations are considered a good sign of fetal health: the fetus is responding to stimuli and displaying integrity of its mechanisms controlling the heart. Accelerations are absent in situations of no fetal movements, e.g. fetal sleep, influence of some drugs, infection and intracerebral haemorrhage. Hence the need for clinical correlation to the CTG findings.

A *deceleration* is a transient episode of slowing of the fetal heart rate below the baseline level of more than 15 bpm and lasting 15 s or more. Decelerations may be greater than this but not significant when other features of the heart rate are normal. The World Health Organization/FIGO definition of duration of a deceleration is 10 s which is too short and includes many normal patterns. When there is an abnormal variability (less than 5 bpm) in a non-reactive trace, decelerations may be very significant even when less than 15 bpm in

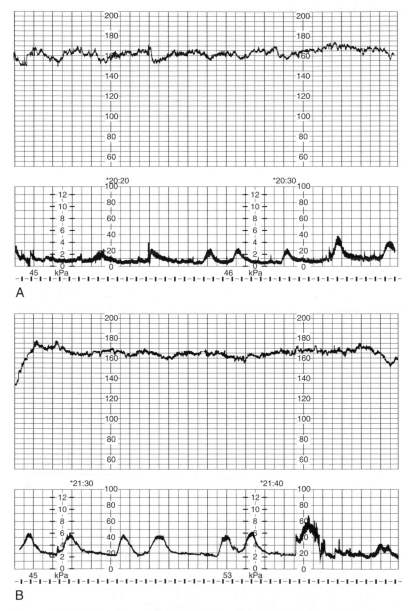

Figure 3.2 (A) Baseline rate 155–160 bpm; (B) rising to 165–170 bpm

amplitude (see later). A deceleration immediately following an acceleration recovering within 30 s is considered normal.

Baseline variability is the degree to which the baseline varies within a particular *band width* excluding accelerations and decelerations (Fig. 3.3). This is a function of the oscillatory amplitude of the baseline. For the purposes of research, oscillatory frequency and oscillatory amplitude may be quantified and scored. This is too complex for routine clinical use and band width is preferred. Figure 3.4 shows band widths classified as reduced (<5 bpm), normal (5–25 bpm) and saltatory (more than 25 bpm).[13] The baseline variability indicates the integrity of the autonomic nervous system. It should be assessed during a reactive period in a 1-min segment showing the greatest band width. Strictly speaking beat-to-beat variation is not seen on traces. The equipment is not designed to analyse every beat interval and uses an averaging technique. In a 1-min interval one cannot see 140 discrete dots. In a research situation beat-to-beat variation can be analysed and is proportionally related to baseline variability. Some workers classify beat-to-beat variation as short-term variability and baseline variability as long-term variability. An understanding of the mechanism of production of baseline variability is crucial to an understanding of fetal heart rate interpretation (see Ch. 4).

Decelerations are *early*, *late* or *variable*. Early decelerations are synchronous with contractions, are usually associated with fetal head

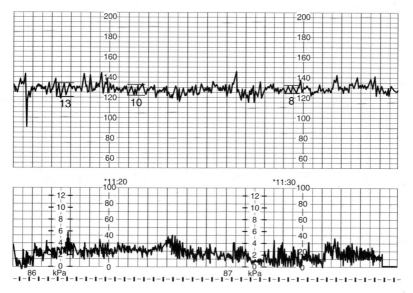

Figure 3.3 Normal band width

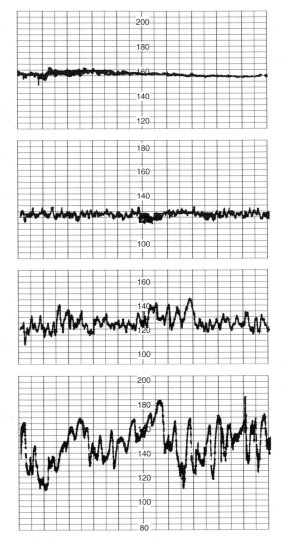

Figure 3.4 Band width classification (reading downwards): silent, hardly any baseline variability (not in the NICE classification but is not a reassuring sign); reduced, <5 bpm; normal, 5–25 bpm; saltatory, over 25 bpm

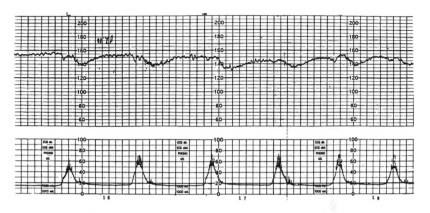

Figure 3.5 Late deceleration

compression and therefore appear in the late first stage and second stage of labour with descent of the head. They are usually, but not invariably, benign. Late decelerations are exactly what their name implies with respect to the contractions. As shown in Figure 3.5 the onset, nadir and recovery are all out of phase with the contraction. They are usually, but not invariably, pathological. The use of the terminology of type I and type II dips does not contribute to further understanding. Variable decelerations vary in shape and sometimes in timing with respect to each other. They may or may not indicate hypoxia. It is critical to evaluate the fetal condition between decelerations and its evolution with time. The integrity of the autonomic control system of the fetal heart must be evaluated (see Ch. 4).

Fetal distress, as implied from a CTG appearance, is not always indicative of hypoxia. Many fetuses are stressed and the challenge is to recognize when this progresses to hypoxic distress. Many babies are delivered operatively for fetal distress (abnormal CTG) and are in excellent condition. This is the crux of the matter in considering the increased caesarean section rate after the introduction of electronic fetal monitoring. We do not *see* fetal distress on a strip of CTG paper. We *see* a fetal heart rate pattern and should describe and classify it as such. It should then be interpreted with respect to the probability of it representing fetal compromise. Anaemia (a low haemoglobin concentration) is not treated rationally without further consideration being given to its aetiology. The same should apply to a fetal heart rate pattern that is not normal. In the light of the clinical situation the likelihood of hypoxia and/or acidosis can be evaluated.

Chapter **4**

Control of the fetal heart and NICE guidelines

Control of the fetal heart is complex (Fig. 4.1). The fetal heart has its own intrinsic activity and a rate determined by the spontaneous activity of the pacemaker in the sinoatrial (SA) node in the atrium. This specialized area of the myocardium initiates the fastest rate and determines the rate in the normal heart. The atrioventricular (AV) node situated on the atrioventricular septum has a slower rate of activity and generates the idioventricular rhythm seen in complete heart block. Under the circumstances of complete heart block the ventricle beats at 60–80 beats per min (bpm).

The fetal heart rate (FHR) is modulated by a number of stimuli. Central nervous system influence is important with cortical and subcortical influences not under voluntary control. We cannot alter our heart rate at will. The cardioregulatory centre in the brain stem also plays a part. Other physiological factors regulate the heart rate such as circulatory catecholamines, chemoreceptors, baroreceptors and their interplay with the autonomic nervous system.[14]

The efferent component of the autonomic nervous system is composed of the sympathetic and parasympathetic systems. There is a constant input from these systems varying from second to second. Sympathetic impulses drive the heart rate to increase while parasympathetic impulses have the opposite effect. If we are confronted with a frightening situation our heart rate involuntarily increases. This puts us under stress, sometimes distress; however, it is an adaptive mechanism preparing us for fright or flight – the sympathetic response. On the contrary, if we are feeling very relaxed and happy at home in the evening after a busy day our heart rate will decrease on account of parasympathetic stimulation.

Electronic FHR monitors compute the heart rate based on averaged intervals between beats extrapolated to what the rate would be if that beat interval remained constant. The machine produces a

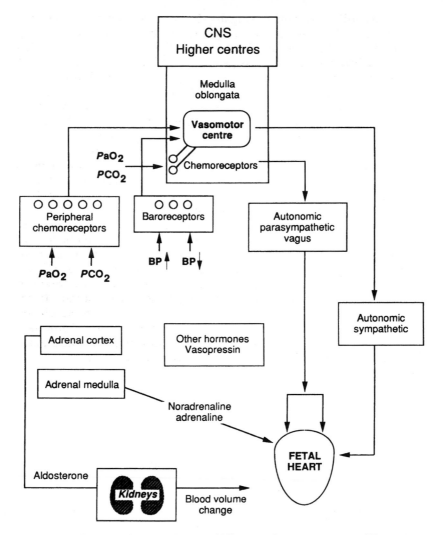

Figure 4.1 Control of the fetal heart. CNS, central nervous system; BP, blood pressure

rate recording after only being applied for a few seconds. However, autonomic impulses immediately and constantly take effect changing the beat intervals and immediately altering the heart rate. This is how baseline variability is generated and it indicates integrity of the autonomic nervous system (Fig. 4.2). Baseline variability is actually seen on the tracing. If it is greatly magnified, individual beats, beat-to-beat variation, can be seen with special equipment used for physiological studies (Fig. 4.3). In practice, baseline variability is the preferred term. The sympathetic nervous system and the parasympathetic or vagal system have the specific effect of generating baseline variability. Suppression of vagal impulses by a drug such as atropine causes tachycardia and reduces baseline variability. Physiological mechanisms are complex and incompletely understood. Fortunately the autonomic nervous system is sensitive to hypoxia at a critical level for the fetus and changes in this response are therefore used as important indicators of wellbeing. The sympathetic and parasympathetic systems mature at slightly different rates with respect to gestational age. The sympathetic system matures faster and this results in marginally faster baseline rates in the preterm period. It is of some interest that male fetuses have slightly faster heart rates than female fetuses, however this is of absolutely no diagnostic value. Before 34 weeks' gestation a higher baseline rate is to be expected. Normal baseline variability suggests good autonomic control and therefore little likelihood of hypoxia.

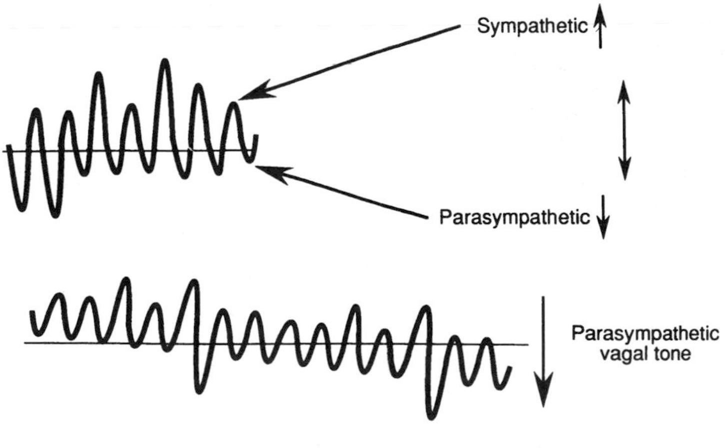

Figure 4.2 Baseline variability: autonomic modulation

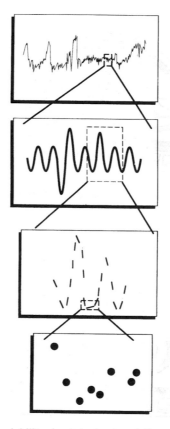

Figure 4.3 Baseline variability: beat-to-beat variation

PATHOPHYSIOLOGICAL MECHANISMS OF DECELERATIONS

An understanding of the maintenance of autonomic control and the mechanisms of decelerations is important. The following illustrations show the effects of contractions on the fetus and blood flow in diagrammatic form (Figs 4.4–4.9).

Early decelerations are early in timing with respect to the uterine contractions and this is therefore a better term than type I dips. They are most commonly due to compression of the fetal head. A rise in intracranial pressure is associated with stimulation of the vagal nerve and bradycardia. This may be caused by a uterine contraction and the sequence of events in this situation is shown in Figures 4.5–4.9. Head compression decelerations are most frequently seen in the late stages of labour when descent of the head is occurring. Indeed, on

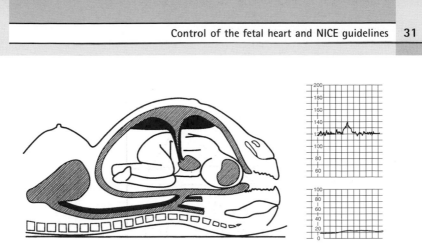

Figure 4.4 Diagrammatic representation of fetus, placenta and blood flow

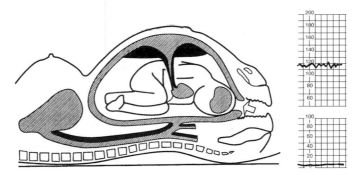

Figure 4.5 Early deceleration: start of contraction

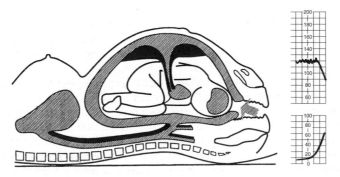

Figure 4.6 Early deceleration: increasing contraction

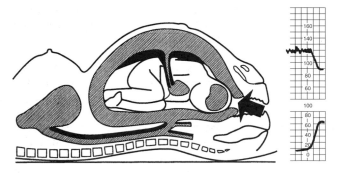

Figure 4.7 Early deceleration: peak of contraction

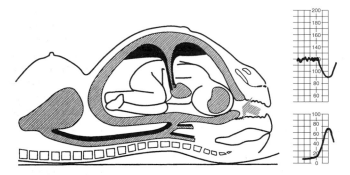

Figure 4.8 Early deceleration: decreasing contraction

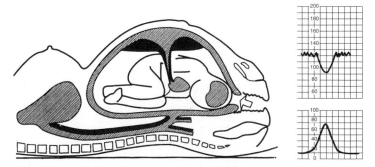

Figure 4.9 Early deceleration: end of contraction

some occasions the onset of the second stage of labour can be deduced from the tracing. Decelerations due to head compression are seen at the time of vaginal examination and also when artificial rupture of the membranes has been performed. Early decelerations with contractions are symmetrical and bell-shaped (Fig. 4.10). The clinical situation should be reviewed to ensure that head compression is a likely explanation at that time. If not, and if the trace is atypical, then an apparently innocuous early deceleration may be an atypical variable deceleration and may be pathological. In one case the obstetric registrar reported that a young West Indian nullipara suffering from sickle cell disease at term but with abdominal size and scan suggesting intrauterine growth restriction was 'niggling' but not yet in established labour. The fetal head was unengaged. He reported the trace (Fig. 4.11) as showing early decelerations. He wished to proceed to induction of labour but the consultant suggested he proceed directly to caesarean section. The registrar was surprised but learned an important lesson on delivering a significantly growth-restricted baby covered in meconium with Apgar scores of 5 and 6 who made a satisfactory recovery. Review of the trace the following day showed that although the decelerations might be described by some as early they do show poor recovery of the second one (atypical variable deceleration), no accelerations and a suggestion of reduced variability after the second deceleration. What is more important is that this fetus had no reason to have head compression and also had a background of risk.

Late decelerations are late in timing with respect to the uterine contraction and are therefore best described as such rather than as type 2 dips. The suggested pathophysiological mechanism of such decelerations is shown in Figures 4.12–4.14. There is a reservoir of

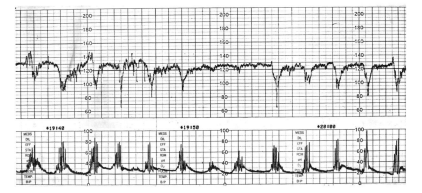

Figure 4.10 Example of early decelerations

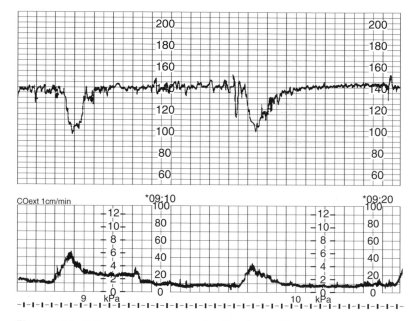

Figure 4.11 Pathological 'early' deceleration (more likely to be atypical variable) – head 4/5 to 5/5 palpable

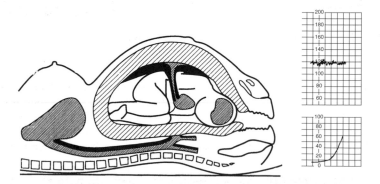

Figure 4.12 Late deceleration: start of contraction

oxygenated blood in the retroplacental space. The size of this space varies and is smaller in intrauterine growth restriction. Poor blood flow to the uteroplacental space is characteristic of fetuses with intra-uterine growth restriction. As a contraction begins the fetus uses up the reservoir of oxygen in the retroplacental space. Due to the restricted supply of blood a hypoxic deceleration begins, it continues through the contraction and does not recover fully until some time

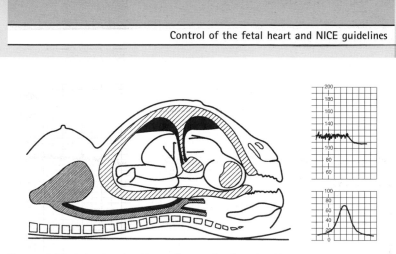

Figure 4.13 Late deceleration: after peak of contraction

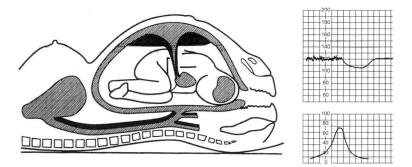

Figure 4.14 Late deceleration: end of contraction

after the contraction when full oxygenation has been restored. The speed of recovery on the ascending limb may reflect the blood flow and the resilience of the fetus. In a non-hypoxic fetus there is increased variability during a deceleration on account of autonomic response. When hypoxia develops there is a tendency to reduced variability.

Baseline variability and decelerations – exception to the rule

A deceleration is defined when the FHR decelerates by more than 15 beats from the baseline for more than 15 s. However, this rule does not apply when the baseline variability is less than 5 beats and any deceleration even less than 15 beats from the baseline could be ominous (Fig. 4.15) unless otherwise proven in a non-reactive trace.

Variable decelerations are the most common type of decelerations and are called variable because they vary in shape, size and sometimes in timing with respect to each other. They vary because they are a manifestation of compression of the umbilical cord and it is

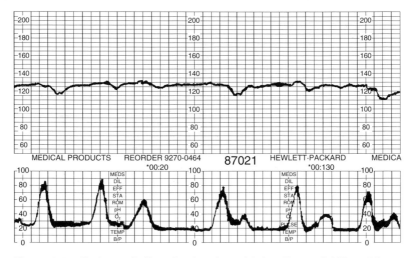

Figure 4.15 Ominous shallow deceleration with baseline variability <5 bpm

compressed in a slightly different way each time. On some occasions it may not be compressed at all and there is no deceleration with that particular contraction. Variable decelerations are more often seen when the amniotic fluid volume is reduced. In North America they are referred to as cord compression decelerations.

The mechanism is illustrated in Figures 4.16–4.20. The umbilical vein has a thinner wall and lower intraluminal pressure than the umbilical arteries (Fig. 4.16). When compression occurs the blood flow through the vein is interrupted before that through the artery. The fetus therefore loses some of its circulating blood volume. When a healthy individual or fetus loses some of its circulating blood volume the natural response effected by the autonomic nervous system is a rise in pulse rate to compensate. A small rise in the FHR therefore appears at the start of a variable deceleration when the fetus is not compromised (Fig. 4.17). After that the umbilical arteries are also occluded, the circulation is relatively restored followed by an increase in systemic pressure, the baroreceptors are stimulated and there is a precipitous fall in the FHR (Fig. 4.18). The deceleration is at its nadir with both vessels occluded. During release of the cord compression arterial flow is restored first with a consequent auto-nomically-mediated sharp rise in heart rate (Fig. 4.19) due to systemic hypotension of blood being pumped out culminating in a small rise in FHR after the deceleration (Fig. 4.20). These rises in FHR before and after decelerations are called shouldering. Whatever they are called, they are a manifestation of a fetus coping well with cord com-pression. The way the cord is being compressed will vary depending

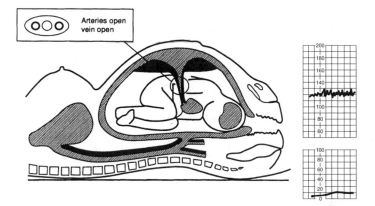

Figure 4.16 Umbilical cord, fetus and placenta: normal circulation

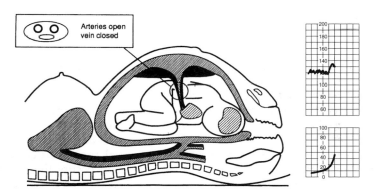

Figure 4.17 Variable deceleration: start of contraction

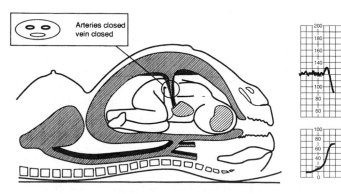

Figure 4.18 Variable deceleration: increasing contraction

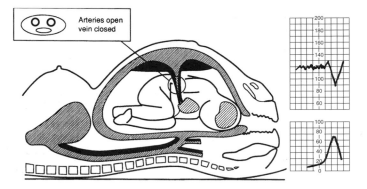

Figure 4.19 Variable deceleration: decreasing contraction

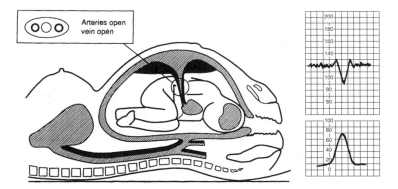

Figure 4.20 Variable deceleration: end of contraction

exactly on how it is positioned with respect to the structure compressing it. On the same basis, variable decelerations may change if the posture of the mother is changed. Normal well-grown fetuses can tolerate cord compression for a considerable length of time before they become hypoxic. Small growth-restricted fetuses do not have the same resilience.

To assess this process it is necessary to analyse the features of the decelerations and also the character of the trace as it evolves. Figure 4.21 shows:

1. normal shouldering
2. exaggeration of shouldering or overshoot (indicates that additional circulations are needed to normalize) which is thought to be prepathological

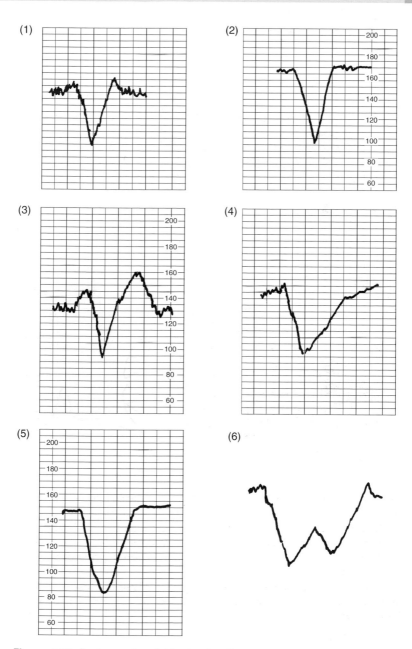

Figure 4.21 Features of variable decelerations

3. loss of shouldering – pathological
4. smoothing of the baseline variability within the deceleration which is associated with loss of variability at the baseline and therefore pathological
5. late recovery – (variable and late deceleration components merged together) has the same pathological significance as late deceleration
6. biphasic deceleration (variable and late decelerations seen as separate components) requiring the same consideration as a late deceleration.

If the duration of the deceleration is more than 60 s and the depth greater than 60 beats, progressive hypoxia becomes more likely.

At times a fetus may have more than one stress operating, e.g. a fetus with intrauterine growth restriction may have cord compression due to oligohydramnios and late decelerations due to reduced amount of retroplacental blood behind the small and partially infarcted placenta. The most critical feature, however, is the evolution of the trace with time. A change in the baseline rate and change in the baseline variability are the key signs of developing hypoxia and acidosis.

Figure 4.22 shows two strips of CTG 60 min apart. In spite of marked variable decelerations, the baseline rate and baseline variability are maintained. So long as adequate progress is being made towards delivery this trace need not cause concern. Figure 4.23 also shows two strips of trace 20 min apart but with quite different features. The progression to a tachycardia with reduced variability suggests developing hypoxia. The time required for a fetus with a previously normal trace to become acidotic related to different patterns of the FHR has been studied.[15] In many cases it may take over 100 min. Medical staff should have time enough to identify the problem and act effectively.

At times it may be difficult to decide whether the decelerations are early, late or variable. It is not only the deceleration itself that is critical but the evolution of the trace with time. The baseline rate between decelerations, the baseline variability and the presence or absence of accelerations are critical.

CLASSIFICATION OF FETAL HEART RATE PATTERN

The NICE guidelines[13] recommend classifying the individual features of baseline rate, baseline variability, decelerations and accelerations as reassuring, non-reassuring or abnormal (Table 4.1), and classifying the whole CTG trace as normal, suspicious or pathological (Box 4.1).

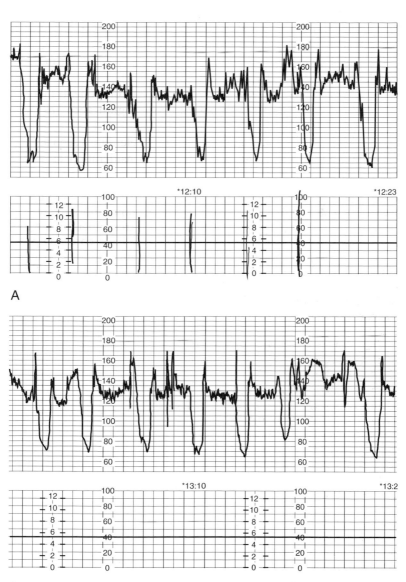

Figure 4.22 Two CTGs recorded 60 min apart, showing variable decelerations. There is no rise in the baseline rate or variability. Occasional decelerations with beat loss >60 and duration >60 secs need close observation.

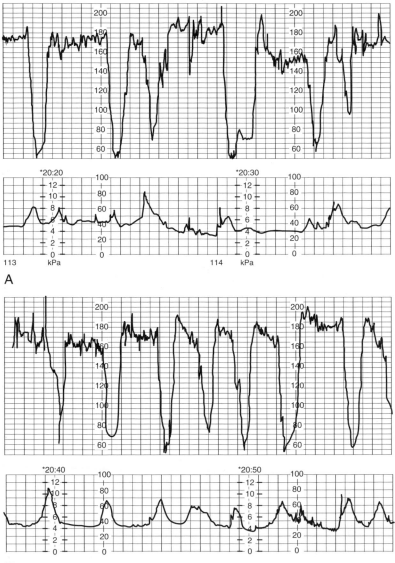

Figure 4.23 Two CTGs recorded 20 min apart. (A) Variable decelerations with abnormal features (duration >60 s, depth >60 beats; tachycardia) (abnormal trace); (B) suggestive of distress (tachycardia and reduced baseline variability)

Table 4.1 Classification of fetal heart rate (FHR) features[a]

Feature	Baseline (bpm)	Variability (bpm)	Decelerations	Accelerations
REASSURING	110–160	≥5	None	Present
NON-REASSURING	100–109 161–180	<5 for 40 to 90 min	Typical variable decelerations with over 50% of contractions, occurring for >90 min Single prolonged deceleration for up to 3 min	The absence of accelerations with an otherwise normal trace is of uncertain significance
ABNORMAL	<100 >180 Sinusoidal pattern ≥10 min	<5 for 90 min	Either atypical variable decelerations with over 50% of contractions or late decelerations, both for over 30 min Single prolonged deceleration for >3 min	

[a] Updated as the book went to press in accordance with NICE Clinical Guideline 55. Intrapartum care: care of healthy women and their babies during childbirth. Issue date September 2007. London: National Institute for Health and Clinical Guidance. Available at www.nice.org.uk/CG055

STOP PRESS: further information about classifying fetal heart rate traces is given on p. 232.

Box 4.1 Cardiotocograph classification

NORMAL – A CTG where all **four** features fall into the reassuring category

SUSPICIOUS – A CTG whose features fall into **one** of the non-reassuring categories and the remainder of the features are reassuring

PATHOLOGICAL – A CTG whose features fall into **two or more** non-reassuring categories or **one or more** abnormal categories

---

A sinusoidal pattern is a regular heart rate with cyclic changes in the FHR baseline like a sine wave, the characteristics of the pattern being that the frequency is less than 6 cycles per min, the amplitude is at least 10 bpm and the duration should be 10 min or longer.

A *normal* classification of the trace implies that the trace assures fetal health. *Suspicious* indicates that continued observation or additional simple tests are required to ensure fetal health. *Pathological* warrants some action in the form of additional tests or delivery depending on the clinical picture. If one of the features of the CTG is abnormal, possible remedial action should be taken and, at times, a short period of observation of the trace may be appropriate if there are no clinical risk factors like intrauterine growth restriction, meconium or infection. If there are clinical risk factors or two abnormal features, additional testing such as fetal scalp blood sampling to elucidate the fetal condition, or delivery, may be more prudent if remedial action does not correct the abnormal features of the trace. If three features of the CTG are abnormal one should consider delivery unless spontaneous delivery is imminent, or perform fetal scalp blood sampling to elucidate the fetal condition. The degree of abnormality of the CTG, clinical risk factors, parity, current cervical dilatation and the rate of progress of labour should determine the decisions to observe, perform a fetal scalp blood sample or deliver promptly.

The expression *fetal distress* should be reconsidered. A trace that is not normal may result from physiological, iatrogenic or pathological causes. The clinical situation and the dynamic evolution of features of the trace with time will clarify the situation.

The underlying principle is to detect fetal compromise using the concept of 'fetal distress' very critically. In all situations, it is consideration of the overall clinical picture that will provide the clues as to whether true fetal compromise is present. Many suspicious CTGs are generated by healthy fetuses demonstrating the ability to respond to stress. For the purposes of clinical decision making, scoring systems or computer analysis have not been found to be useful particularly in the intrapartum period.

Chapter 5

Cardiotocographic interpretation: the basics

A fetal heart rate (FHR) trace has four easily definable features: baseline rate, baseline variability, accelerations and decelerations. The baseline rate (normal 110–160 beats per min (bpm)) is identified by drawing a line through the midpoint of the 'wiggliness' which represents the most common rate, having excluded accelerations and decelerations. The baseline variability (normal 5–25 bpm) is determined by drawing horizontal lines at the level of the highest point of the peak and lowest point of the troughs of the 'wiggliness' of the trace in a 1-cm segment (Fig. 5.1).

The dynamic state of the fetal cardiovascular system and the concept of fetal behavioural state must be appreciated. Fetuses that have a neurologically normal behavioural state have quiet sleep periods associated with rapid eye movements, and active sleep periods without such movements. Active movements are associated with good variability and accelerations. Quiet sleep is associated with episodes of decreased variability which generally last for up to 40 min. This phenomenon of active and quiet epochs that alternate is known as 'cycling'. Interpretation of a trace as normal is absolutely dependent on recognition of this physiological phenomenon. Absence of cycling may be due to hypoxia, infection, medication (e.g. sedatives), recreational drugs, maternal anaesthesia, fetal brain haemorrhage or major fetal neurological malformation.

Baseline variability is best interpreted during the active phase, recognized by the presence of accelerations defined as rises of 15 beats or more from the baseline lasting for 15 s or more. The presence of two accelerations in a 20-min trace is termed a reactive trace and is suggestive of a fetus in good health. The accelerations usually coincide with fetal movements reflecting the activity of the 'somatic' nervous system. These fetuses usually have normal baseline FHR variability. A trace can be described as reactive within a short time once a normal baseline rate, normal baseline variability

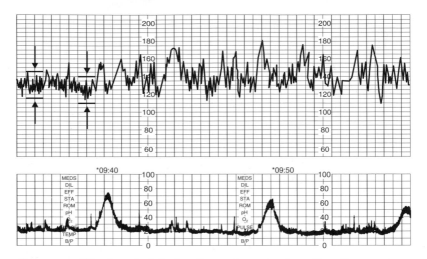

Figure 5.1 'Wiggliness' of the baseline – determination of baseline variability (best segment representative of autonomic nervous system activity to be chosen)

and accelerations are identified. This will indicate a non-hypoxic fetus. Absence of decelerations in the presence of contractions would indicate that there is no stress of cord compression or reduced retroplacental reserve. However, in order to be described as non-reactive it should run for a period of at least 40 min during which two accelerations are not identified in any 20-min period. FHR decelerations signify a transient event. Early decelerations in the late first stage and early second stage of labour generally indicate head compression and rarely compromise. Late decelerations indicate transient hypoxia with impaired uteroplacental perfusion which may proceed to established acidosis. Variable decelerations are often due to cord compression but are also seen in fetuses in breech presentation and occipitoposterior position when the postulated mechanism is pressure on the supraorbital region of the head. Developing hypoxia and acidosis are suggested by the absence of accelerations, a rise in the baseline rate and a reduction in baseline variability.

Accelerations are the hallmark of fetal health.

Features of a reactive trace are shown in Figure 5.2. In looking at this trace think of a child playing in a field. The child has a normal pulse rate (baseline rate), minor movements of the limbs suggestive of activity (good baseline variability) and is tossing a ball up and down (accelerations). If the child is tired or is unwell it will start restricting its activity and stop tossing the ball (absence of accelera-

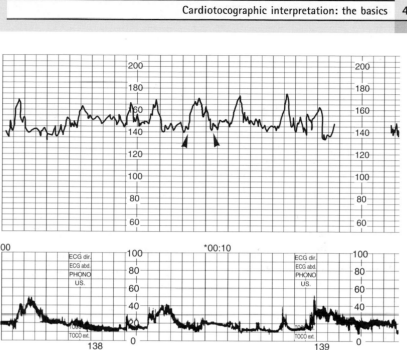

Figure 5.2 Reactive trace – two accelerations in 20 min

tions is the first thing to be noticed when hypoxia develops suggesting that either the child is not well or is tired). Then the child would either sit or lie down to rest. In such a situation it is difficult to differentiate healthy tiredness from impending sickness. A persistently raised pulse rate after a period of rest would suggest the latter (baseline tachycardia). The fetus has limited capacity to respond to hypoxia by increasing its cardiac stroke volume and has to increase its cardiac output by an increase in heart rate. Reduction in baseline variability and finally a flat baseline are the progressive features with increasing hypoxia. This is analogous to a rapid thready pulse in a sick person and should be borne in mind when analysing traces. The baseline variability is due to the sympathetic and parasympathetic activities. An injection of atropine to the mother will increase the FHR and abolish the variability due to the abolition of the parasympathetic activity.

Figure 5.3 shows a reactive trace with accelerations, normal rate, normal variability but a section of the trace was not registered. In the segment after the missing portion there are no accelerations, normal rate but reduced baseline variability. A child who was in good health a few minutes ago cannot suddenly become sick without an obvious reason. The absence of accelerations and reduced baseline variability

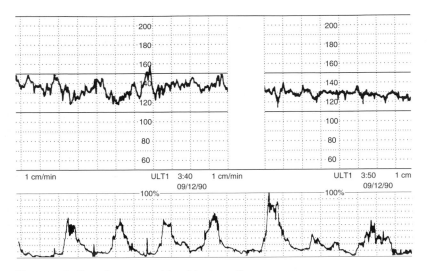

Figure 5.3 Reactive trace with a blank section

suggest that the fetus is in the quiet phase. This interpretation is further strengthened because there is no increase in the baseline FHR. There are contractions present but no corresponding decelerations. This indicates that there is no stress to the fetus such as cord compression or reduction in retroplacental pool of blood that may cause hypoxia. In labour evolution of hypoxia is 'unlikely' without decelerations.

Figure 5.4 shows a trace with a baseline FHR of 120 bpm with normal baseline variability and an isolated deceleration followed by marked accelerations. The normal baseline rate and variability with marked accelerations (tossing the ball up and down) suggest that the fetus is not hypoxic. The isolated deceleration may be due to brief cord compression associated with fetal movement. In the intrapartum situation this may be accounted for by fetal movements, uterine contractions or reduced amniotic fluid due to the membranes having ruptured. This is not an immediate threat to the fetus but further continuous electronic fetal monitoring is indicated. In the antenatal period the possibility of reduced amniotic fluid has to be considered either due to intrauterine growth restriction, prelabour rupture of the membranes or postmaturity. Ultrasound evaluation should be undertaken. If the amniotic fluid volume is normal the deceleration may be due to pressure on the cord due to fetal movement.

Figure 5.5 shows a trace with repetitive variable decelerations. At the beginning of the trace the baseline rate is 120 bpm, there are no

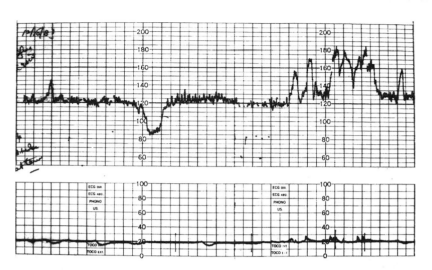

Figure 5.4 Reactive trace with isolated deceleration

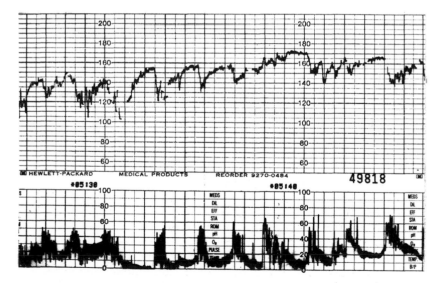

Figure 5.5 Repetitive variable decelerations – developing asphyxia

accelerations and the baseline variability is normal. Towards the end of the trace the baseline rate has risen to 160 bpm with decrease in baseline variability. This suggests an attempt to compensate in response to the evolving hypoxia.

PAPER SPEED

It is important to check the paper speed of any cardiotocograph (CTG) tracing before interpretation. It is not easy for someone who is trained to interpret traces at 1 cm/min to interpret a trace recorded at a speed of 3 cm/min. With current fetal monitoring technology the paper speed is annotated automatically on the trace. If the paper speed is not annotated on the trace, scrutiny of the contraction duration would give a clue that the paper speed is more than 1 cm/min as the contraction duration on the trace would be 2–3 min which is an unlikely event in normal labour. Figure 5.6 shows the effect on the trace by changing paper speed during the recording. Figure 5.7 shows comparative traces recorded at different paper speeds. At the faster paper speed features such as baseline variability, accelerations and decelerations are altered. The baseline variability appears more reduced than actually is the case, accelerations are difficult to identify (Fig. 5.7A and B), and the decelerations appear to be of a longer duration (Fig. 5.6). It is the practice in the UK, some European countries

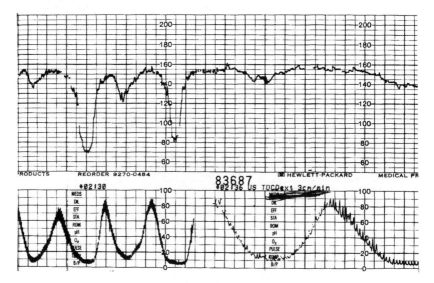

Figure 5.6 Changing paper speed during recording

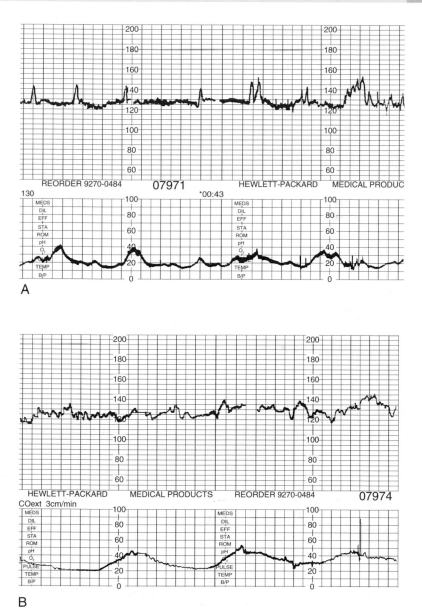

Figure 5.7 Two recordings from the same patient at (A) 1 cm/min; (B) 3 cm/min

and in Asia to use a paper speed of 1 cm/min (thus reducing the number of trees being cut down to produce paper), while practitioners in the USA run the paper at 3 cm/min. For a trained eye the paper speed does not matter, but for day-to-day interpretation it is better to have the paper speed at the rate the staff is used to – failure to appreciate this has led to confusion and serious error. The current fetal monitors have their paper speed switch mechanism either behind the paper loading tray which has to be removed to alter the paper speed or in a position so that it is difficult to alter the speed accidentally. Although the discussion on paper speed may appear trivial, failure to recognize the difference has resulted in unnecessary caesarean sections both in the antenatal and intrapartum periods. Such simple mistakes expose the mother to an unnecessary anaesthetic and surgical risk and put her at high risk in her next pregnancy.

PROBLEMS ASSOCIATED WITH THE INTERPRETATION OF BASELINE VARIABILITY

Any FHR tracing has periods of high and low baseline variability cycles both in the antenatal and intrapartum periods. These periods of 'silent phase' with low baseline variability can be as short as 7–10 min in the antenatal period and from 25–40 min in the intrapartum period.[16,17] Although baseline variability can be referred to at any given point in the trace, the health of the baby is best judged when the trace is reactive (i.e. when the baby is active and 'playing with the ball' rather than when the baby is sleeping). It is similar to us being judged at an interview when we are active and awake rather than inactive and sleeping.

Reduced baseline variability

The commonest reasons for reduced baseline variability are:

1. the 'sleep' or 'quiet' phase of the FHR cycle (Fig. 5.8)
2. hypoxia
3. prematurity
4. tachycardia (>180 bpm – due to technical issues)
5. drugs (sedatives, antihypertensives acting on CNS and anaesthetics)
6. congenital malformation (of the central nervous system more commonly than the cardiovascular system)
7. cardiac arrhythmias

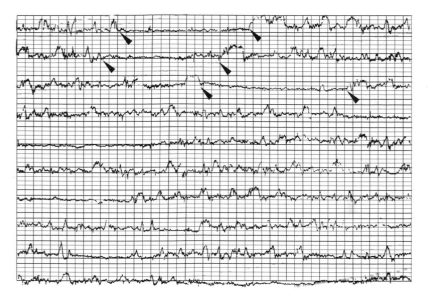

Figure 5.8 Composite trace. Reduced baseline variability: period of fetal 'sleep' alternating with 'active' periods

8. fetal anaemia (Rhesus disease or fetomaternal haemorrhage)
9. fetal infection.

High and low variability cycles ('cycling')

When a trace is seen with reduced baseline variability (band width <5 bpm), the previous segments of the trace must be reviewed. If the preceding trace was reactive with good baseline variability, then the segment being reviewed is probably in the 'quiet phase' of the baby's FHR cycle and there is no cause for alarm. The start of another active cycle can be awaited especially if there have been no decelerations or increases in the baseline rate which might indicate the possibility of hypoxia. If there was no previous segment of the trace to consider, the clinical picture must be reviewed to identify whether the fetus is at risk (e.g. small fundosymphysis height, post-term, thick meconium, no or scanty amniotic fluid at the time of membrane rupture, reduced fetal movements, other obstetric risk factors) or is influenced by medication (e.g. pethidine, antihypertensives, etc.) at the same time continuing the trace when reactivity with good baseline variability may appear.

Pethidine and baseline variability

Sometimes there is concern about giving pethidine to women in labour in case it reduces the baseline variability and obscures the reduced baseline variability of hypoxia. Before giving pethidine it is important to make sure the FHR trace is reactive and normal with no evidence of hypoxia. Once the pethidine is given the accelerations may not be evident and the baseline variability may become reduced as in the 'quiet' or 'sleep' phase. The period of this quiet phase following pethidine in some fetuses can extend beyond the natural quiet phase expected and thus leads to anxiety. In labour, if the trace has been reactive and the fetus was not hypoxic, hypoxia can develop only gradually due to regular uterine contractions cutting off the blood supply to the placenta, unless acute events such as abruption, cord prolapse, scar dehiscence or oxytocic hyperstimulation occur. Alternatively, it can be due to cord compression with each contraction. The reduction of blood supply to the retroplacental area by regular uterine contractions will present with late decelerations, and that due to cord compression will present with variable decelerations. If these are affecting the fetus and causing hypoxia, the fetus tends to compensate for the hypoxia by increasing the cardiac output, which it does by increasing the FHR as it has limited capacity to increase the stroke volume. Therefore, if the FHR pattern after pethidine does not show any decelerations and no increase in the baseline rate, despite the fact that there are no accelerations and the baseline variability is reduced, these features are likely to be due to pethidine rather than to hypoxia. When the baby is born, the baby may not cry and may need stimulation or reversal of drug effect by Naloxone or assisted ventilation because of the effect of the drug on the central nervous system causing respiratory depression, but the neonate will have good cord arterial blood status indicating that there was no intrauterine hypoxia.

False baseline variability due to technical reasons

Modern machines have autocorrelation and do not pose technical problems related to baseline variability but the older machines did not have autocorrelation and gave a false impression of exaggerated baseline variability when the FHR was recorded using an ultrasound transducer. Although one may not encounter this in current practice, traces from several years ago may be brought up to you for medicolegal reasons and hence the explanation is offered in this section.

The baseline variability seen on the trace is produced by the time differences between individual heart beats. One segment of the serration or undulation, i.e. one upswing which contributes to baseline variability, is only a few millimetres but is representative of a number of beats, as outlined earlier. The machine calculates the beat intervals from the impulses coming back to the transducer which arise from the movements of the fetal heart. However, there may be extraneous impulses from other sources (caused by movement of the bowel or of the anterior abdominal wall of the mother) which may be misinterpreted and a falsely exaggerated baseline variability produced (Fig. 5.9). When the fetus becomes hypoxic, usually the first feature to be observed is the disappearance of the accelerations, followed by an increase in baseline FHR and a reduction in the baseline variability. In Figure 5.9, there is tachycardia, with a FHR of 160 bpm, there are no accelerations and there are variable decelerations suggestive of possible fetal compromise. This was from a growth-restricted fetus with little amniotic fluid surrounding it. The other features on the trace (absence of accelerations, tachycardia and decelerations) are not consistent with the 'good baseline variability' observed on the trace. The problem is that the trace was obtained on a fetal monitor without autocorrelation facilities. The baseline variability obtained on the ultrasound mode with the old fetal monitors is not reliable and in labour it is best to use a scalp electrode with these machines. Figure 5.10 shows an abnormal trace with tachycardia, no accelerations and with reduced variability. The switch from ultrasound to direct electrocardiograph (ECG) mode gives the markedly reduced (flat) true baseline variability of the sick fetus. Using modern machines should obviate this problem (Fig. 5.11).

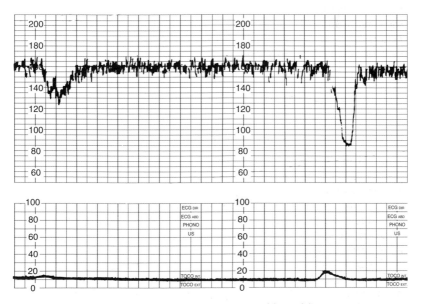

Figure 5.9 Artefactual variability due to old machine without autocorrelation facility

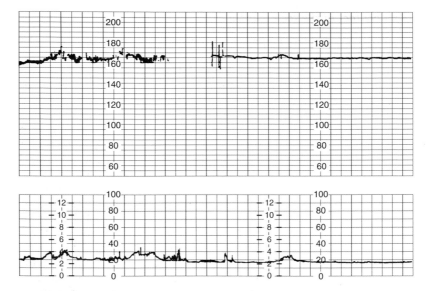

Figure 5.10 Artefactual variability obscuring pathological trace rectified by using scalp electrode

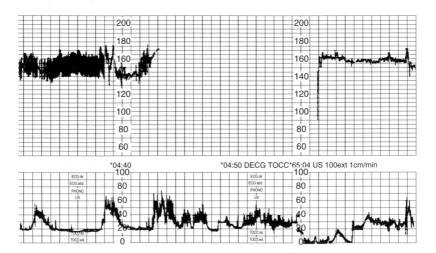

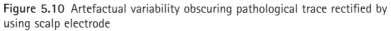

Figure 5.11 Effect on variability of changing monitoring mode from fetal electrode to ultrasound in a machine with autocorrelation facility

Poor contact of the scalp electrode

'Picket fence' artefact is not an uncommon problem with the use of scalp electrodes (Fig. 5.12). The vertical deviation of the baseline, unlike the undulations, suggests that it is artefact. Figure 5.13 shows a baseline tachycardia with a rate of 150 bpm. There are no accelerations and careful attention reveals that the baseline variability is markedly reduced (less than 5 bpm) and is masked by artefact. This is usually thought to be due to poor contact of the electrode with fetal tissue or the absence of proper contact of the reference electrode (a metal piece at the base of the electrode) to maternal tissue. Although replacing the electrode and applying an adhesive skin electrode to the maternal thigh as a reference electrode may be of some help, usually these manoeuvres do not markedly improve the quality of the recording. In these situations it is better to record the FHR tracing with an external ultrasound transducer which has autocorrelation facilities. These fetal monitors give a good quality trace with a baseline variability which is equivalent to that which can be obtained with a scalp electrode. In the past, when a good quality trace was not obtained with external ultrasound transducers, the use of internal electrodes was advocated, whereas currently the use of external ultrasound transducers is indicated when the FHR trace with an internal electrode is not satisfactory (see Fig. 5.11). Because of the good quality tracing obtained with fetal monitors using autocorrelation technol-

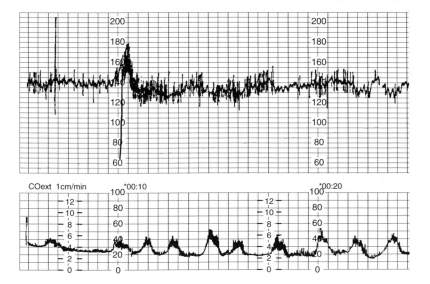

Figure 5.12 'Picket fence' artefact due to poor contact of fetal electrode

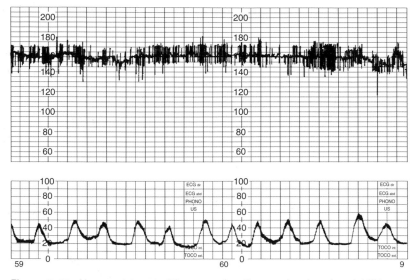

Figure 5.13 Abnormal trace with no accelerations and reduced variability being hidden by 'picket fence' artefact

ogy, there is no necessity to rupture the membranes in labour in order to place an electrode. The indications for artificial rupture of the membranes are during augmentation of slow labour and to inspect the colour of the amniotic fluid when a trace is abnormal. The 'picket fence' artefact can rarely be due to cardiac arrhythmias, and it may be useful to obtain the actual ECG signals from the fetal monitor. This can be obtained on the CTG chart paper with some machines (Fig. 5.14), or it can be obtained by connecting a lead to a conventional ECG machine from an outlet in the back of the fetal monitor. If the 'picket fencing' has a regular pattern and the distance above and below the baseline is nearly equal throughout the trace then it may be due to cardiac arrhythmia. If not, it is likely to be a problem with disturbance in the signal-to-noise ratio due to the electrode.

Other interference

Extraneous electrical influences can produce artefact in the baseline variability and if the disturbance exceeds the frequency of signals obtained from the FHR using a scalp electrode it can completely confuse the FHR signals with no FHR tracing. The use of transcutaneous electrical nerve stimulation (TENS) or the obstetric pulsar used for pain relief can produce this problem, and Figure 5.15 illustrates this with FHR tracing and the corresponding ECG signals.

With TENS external ultrasound monitoring is preferable.

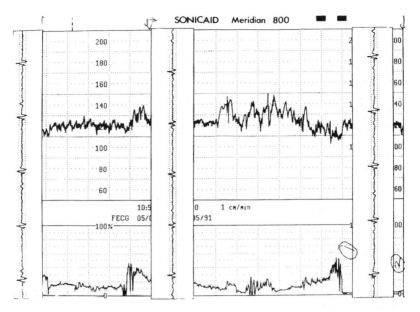

Figure 5.14 ECG signals on CTG

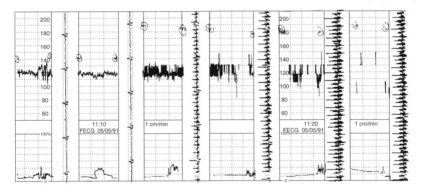

Figure 5.15 Effect of TENS on the trace as the TENS frequency rate is increased

CORRECT IDENTIFICATION OF BASELINE HEART RATE

Persistent accelerations may lead to confusion such that some traces have been termed 'pseudodistress' patterns. When the fetus is very active it may show so many accelerations that it is misinterpreted as tachycardia with decelerations (Fig. 5.16). This situation can arise in the antenatal period or in labour. Certain clues aid correct interpreta-

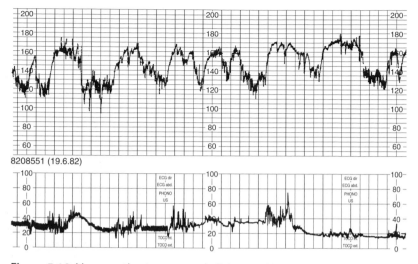

Figure 5.16 Very reactive trace: pseudodistress pattern

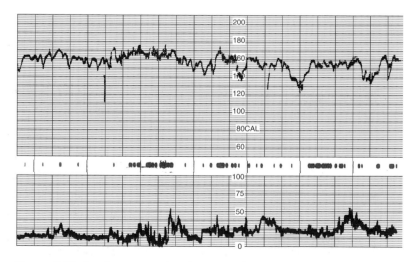

Figure 5.17 Continuous accelerations: very frequent use of event marker

tion. The clinical picture and risk assessment will indicate the probability of true compromise. Figures 5.17 and 5.18 show greater degrees of the same phenomenon and are more difficult to interpret. The trace may appear to show a long period of tachycardia and confluent accelerations. In the antenatal period, it is easier to recognize these patterns as non-pathological if the fetus is well grown, has a normal

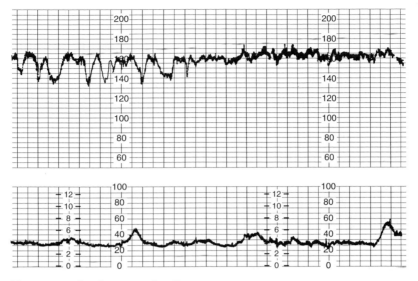

Figure 5.18 Confluent accelerations

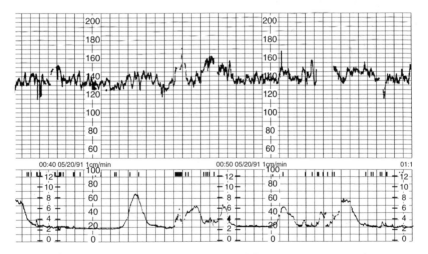

Figure 5.19 Hewlett-Packard 1350 with a combi transducer; automatic fetal movement recording through the ultrasound channel

amniotic fluid volume and is moving actively during the recording of the trace. This will be most obviously demonstrated by frequent use of the event marker by the mother or by evidence of fetal movements on the tocography channel (see Fig. 5.17). Many fetal monitors detect fetal movements automatically (Fig. 5.19). Such traces should have good baseline variability both at the true rate and at the higher rate. The true baseline rate on these traces is not below 110 bpm (the lower limit of normal for a healthy fetus). Inspection of the trace prior to the segment where there is doubt as to the true baseline rate would provide evidence of the true baseline rate. If such a segment is not available, continuation of the trace for a longer period should provide it. Repeatedly in clinical practice this pattern is misunderstood resulting in unnecessary intervention and the birth of a vigorous neonate behaving after delivery as it did before: Apgar scores of 9 and 10 after a caesarean section for 'fetal distress'.

A hypoxic fetus with a tachycardia with or without decelerations does not move actively.

At times there may be difficulty in resolving this issue. Figure 5.20a may be considered to show stress or a very active fetus. The tocography channel suggests rather frequent contractions, and after the reduction in the rate of oxytocin and contraction frequency a more understandable picture emerges (Fig. 5.20b). Further evaluation may be necessary with biophysical assessment antenatally or fetal scalp blood sampling intrapartum. If an oxytocin infusion is in progress its rate should be reduced.

Importance of recognition of the baseline heart rate for each fetus

When a fetus is in good health the baseline FHR tends to vary by 10–15 bpm in an undulating way, slowing slightly in the sleep phase and after maternal sedation. It rises slightly during the active phase when the fetus moves, exhibiting a number of accelerations. Gradually increasing hypoxia causes the FHR to rise gradually to a tachycardia. During the evolution of persistent repetitive decelerations recognition of the steadily rising baseline rate due to compensation potentially leading to compromise is important. Each fetus has its own baseline rate and, although it may still be within the normal range, for that individual fetus it can represent a significant rise. It is important to take note of the baseline rate at the beginning of the trace and to compare it with the current rate. In the antenatal period comparison of the baseline heart rate of sequential traces has the same relevance. Priority should be given to the revised definition of normal baseline FHR, 110–160 bpm, bearing these considerations in mind. Any tracing with a baseline rate of greater than 160 bpm should be carefully scrutinized for other suspicious features. Traces within the normal range for baseline rate may be abnormal or ominous on account of other features (Fig. 5.21).

A normal baseline rate can be associated with hypoxia and an ominous trace.

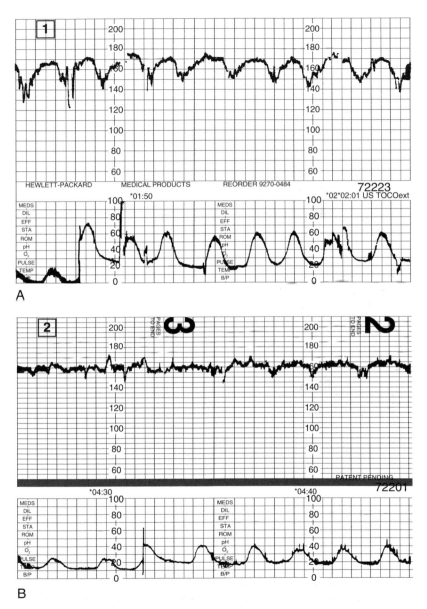

Figure 5.20 Trace showing (A) hyperstimulation and tachycardia; (B) followed by reduction of oxytocin and resolution

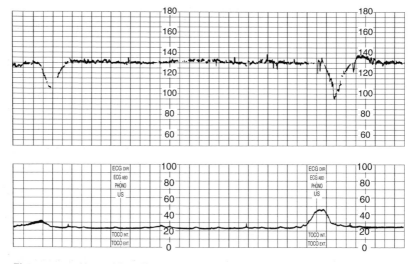

Figure 5.21 Normal baseline rate: pathological trace, with no accelerations, reduced baseline variability ('silent pattern') and shallow late decelerations

Baseline tachycardia and bradycardia

A range of 160–180 bpm is termed a *baseline tachycardia* and a range of 100–110 bpm is called *baseline bradycardia*. Although they are categorized in the suspicious category in the NICE guidelines, provided there is good baseline variability, accelerations and the absence of decelerations these FHRs do not generally represent hypoxia. Figure 5.22 shows a moderate baseline tachycardia but other features are reassuring.

Figure 5.23 is a rare trace showing sinus bradycardia at 80 bpm with a trace otherwise remarkably normal. The baby was born in good condition with a good outcome. The mother had had a renal transplant and was taking various medications including beta-blockers for hypertension.

Tachycardia

Tachycardia with a baseline rate of greater than 160 bpm should prompt a search for other suspicious features such as absence of accelerations, poor baseline variability and decelerations. Tachycardia is not uncommon in preterm fetuses due to earlier maturation of the sympathetic nervous system. With increasing maturity of the fetus the baseline heart rate gradually falls and at term is often

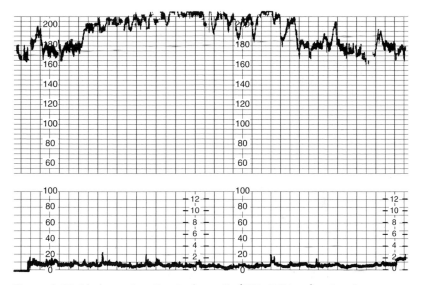

Figure 5.22 Moderate baseline tachycardia (150–170 bpm); other features are reassuring

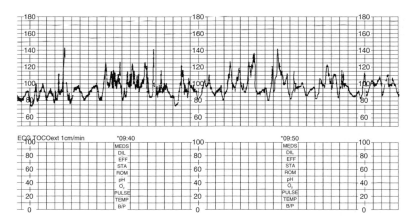

Figure 5.23 Sinus bradycardia

between 110 and 140 bpm. Fetal tachycardia may be due to fetal movement or increased sympathetic tone caused by arousal associated with noise, pain or acoustic stimulation. Fetal hypoxia, hypovolaemia and anaemia are pathological causes of tachycardia. Maternal sympathomimetic activation due to pain or anxiety may lead to fetal tachycardia, as can dehydration leading to poor uterine perfusion.

Pain relief, reassurance and hydration may be expected to reverse this. Administration of betamimetic drugs to inhibit preterm labour increases sympathetic activity, whereas anticholinergic drugs such as atropine abolish parasympathetic activity through the vagal nerve resulting in tachycardia.

False or erroneous baseline FHR because of scale differences

In general, electronic fetal monitors accept paper of about the same width; however, paper has been manufactured with different scales. In the UK machines have been calibrated to an expected paper display of 50–210 bpm with a 20 bpm per cm scale sensitivity. It is important that this be uniform so that observers' perception of rate and variability is not compromised. Technically this could be solved by the manufacturers standardizing the aspect ratio irrespective of size of paper and paper speed.

False or erroneous baseline because of double counting of low baseline FHR

In normal circumstances the atrium and ventricle beat almost simultaneously followed by the next complete cardiac movement of the atrium and ventricle. The reflected ultrasound from these two chambers or even from one of the walls (atrium, ventricle or the valves) is used by the machine to compute the FHR. When the FHR is slow, at 70–80 bpm, there is a longer time interval between the atrial and the ventricular contractions. The machine recognizes each of the reflected sounds (one from the ventricle and the other from the atrium) as two separate beats and computes the rate, which may mimic the FHR as it will be in the expected range for a normal fetal heart. For most observers the sound generated will also give an impression that the FHR is within the normal range; this is because the heart sounds from the machine are always the same for every baby – they are electronic noise. During the false counting or 'doubling' of the FHR episode, listening with a fetal stethoscope will reveal the true situation. The suspicion that something is amiss will be aroused by the FHR tracing, which may show a steady baseline of 140 bpm but at times will be 70 bpm. Because it is a double counting phenomenon the upper rate on the recording paper will be exactly double that of the lower rate and can be easily checked by auscultation. Such a trace can also be due to the machine recognizing an atrial rate of 140 bpm and a ventricular rate of 70 bpm at different times in a case with complete heart block (Fig. 5.24). The mother may have an autoimmune disorder. Doubling the rate is a phenomenon dependent on the use of ultrasound monitoring. A fetal electrode will not show this effect and should therefore be used if in doubt. A situation of bradycardia with

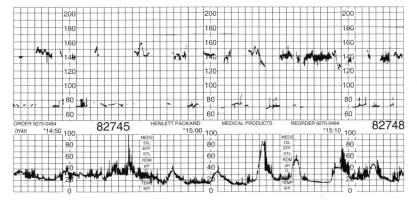

Figure 5.24 Intermittent double counting: heart block in maternal systemic lupus erythematosus

the doubling effect may be observed in a sick fetus as an acute episode and a preterminal event.

Beware of double counting.

Bradycardia: fetal or maternal?

There is a facility, not well known and not commonly used, to record the maternal heart rate by using the external ECG mode of the monitor by applying skin electrodes, supplied with the equipment, to the maternal chest. The trace obtained is identical to fetal recordings (Fig. 5.25), particularly when maternal anxiety or betamimetic therapy for preterm labour results in a maternal tachycardia. If the woman reports with reduced fetal movements she may have a tachycardia due to anxiety, and this may be mistaken for the actual FHR while the fetus is dead. Note that the lower trace, which is maternal, accelerates and has variability as does the fetal trace.

Always use the fetal stethoscope before applying the machine. This is the advice of the Medical Devices Agency of the UK.

When the fetus is dead the ultrasound may be inadvertently directed at maternal vessels. The technical quality of this trace is usually poor with incomplete continuity. In such circumstances it is prudent to verify the presence of the fetal heart activity by auscultation, confirming with an ultrasound scan if there is doubt.

If two baseline rates appear which do not show the 'doubling' phenomenon the transducer may be picking up the fetal heart at one time and the maternal pulse at another time. The trace in Figure 5.26 was recorded in preterm labour treated with betamimetic drugs showing fetal and maternal tachycardia. This should be verified by

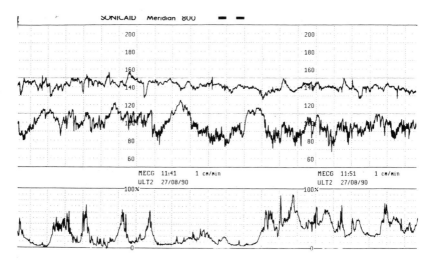

Figure 5.25 Fetal (upper) and maternal (lower) trace recording

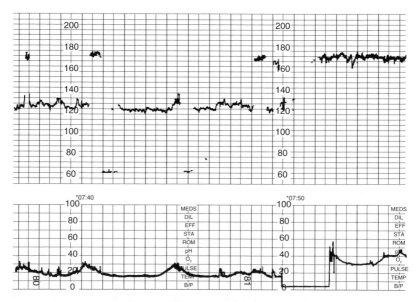

Figure 5.26 Maternal (120 bpm) and fetal (170 bpm) tachycardia: ultrasound mode

counting the maternal pulse at the wrist and by auscultating the fetal heart simultaneously. The findings should be documented on the CTG paper for clinical and medico-legal purposes.

Fetal arrhythmia

Complete fetal heart block may be recorded as a stable bradycardia and may give a trace as shown in Figure 5.24. Incomplete heart block is more of a dilemma. Both diagnoses should be substantiated by a detailed B-mode ultrasound scan and further investigation. A heart block must be a proportion of the actual rate (2:1, 3:1) and this should be analysed. Confirmed heart block should prompt a search in the mother's blood for autoimmune antibodies even if she is asymptomatic. Fetal heart block compromises intrapartum surveillance and alternative methods to electronic fetal monitoring should be used (clinical sense, fetal blood sampling, Doppler blood flow study).

Occasional dropped beats or ectopic beats are a relatively common phenomenon in normal fetuses, however more persistent arrhythmias can be associated with hypoxia.

PROBLEMS ASSOCIATED WITH INTERPRETATION OF TRACES

In the past much time and effort has been spent on categorizing decelerations into 'early', 'late' and 'variable', rather than interpreting the trace as a whole in relation to the clinical situation. A given trace may be acceptable as normal in the late first stage but not in the early first stage of labour. At times it is difficult to classify the decelerations as early, variable or late. Often they may have mixed features of variable and late decelerations. It is far more important to categorize any trace as normal, suspicious or pathological. The NICE recommendations for the classification of the features of the CTG and the CTG as a whole have been described in Chapter 4.

Figure 5.27 shows a trace with tachycardia, no accelerations, reduced baseline variability and repetitive decelerations. Clinically the fetus is post-term and the mother is in early labour. This is a grossly abnormal trace demanding intervention. The decelerations may be analysed as variable because of the precipitous fall in the baseline rate characteristic of cord compression and because the decelerations vary in shape and size. They may be considered to be late because of the lateness in recovery. However, even when the decelerations are ignored the trace is abnormal because there are no accelerations, the baseline rate is greater than 160 bpm and the baseline variability is less than 5 bpm. There should be no hesitation in classifying this trace as pathological. Those who have limited knowledge of the pathophysiology of FHR may spend time arguing about

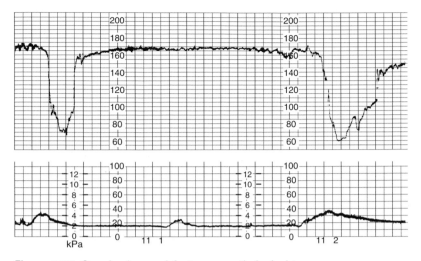

Figure 5.27 Grossly abnormal features – pathological trace

the nature of the decelerations without concentrating on the whole trace and the clinical picture.

Intervention is mandatory.

Figure 5.28 shows a pathological trace but this is difficult to recognize unless one is aware of the exception to the rule of interpreting FHR traces. The rate can be within the normal range (110–160 bpm) but with reduced baseline variability (<5 bpm) and repeated late decelerations less than 15 bpm. This is an ominous picture unless the trace has shown recent reactive segments. The clinical picture has to be considered and, at times, an immediate delivery is opted for on clinical grounds. All the features of a given trace must be considered before it is categorized as normal, suspicious or pathological. The subsequent management of patients depends on this.

Shallow decelerations with reduced baseline variability in the 'quiet epoch' following an 'active epoch' with accelerations have been found to be associated with fetal breathing episodes.[18] If, on admission or commencement of the CTG, there is reduced baseline variability and shallow decelerations, one should look for clinical symptoms and signs that might suggest possible hypoxia or other insults, e.g. reduced or absent fetal movements, infection, intrauterine growth restriction, prolonged pregnancy and vaginal bleeding. If no such symptoms or signs are evident but mother is at, or close to, term and is in early labour, artificial rupture of membranes may reveal thick meconium with scanty fluid highlighting possible compromise and the need for delivery. In the absence of the above and the baseline variability is >5 bpm, or at least 3–5 bpm, it may be

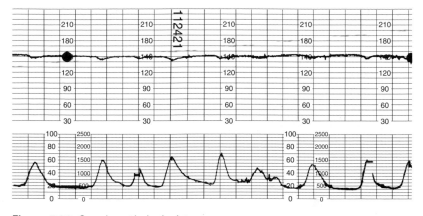

Figure 5.28 Grossly pathological trace

acceptable to wait for up to 40 and a maximum of 90 min for the next active epoch with accelerations to become evident. If facilities permit, use of an ultrasound to observe the quantity of liquor, fetal body or breathing movements and fetal tone may be useful. If it is in the antenatal period and the fetus is preterm it may be prudent to undertake the above biophysical assessment and also to determine fetal growth and examine the blood flow in the umbilical arteries and the fetal vessels. If these facilities or expertise are not available consideration should be given for delivery based on the clinical features and fetal maturity.

- Accelerations and normal baseline variability are the hallmarks of fetal health.
- A hypoxic fetus can have a normal baseline rate, other features being abnormal.
- In the absence of accelerations, repeated shallow decelerations (below 15 bpm) are ominous when baseline variability is less than 5 bpm.

Chapter 6

Antepartum fetal surveillance

Antenatal care should be appropriate and effective. The low-risk mother will be seen largely by the midwife in community antenatal clinics. Higher-risk mothers will be seen in hospital antenatal clinics often by doctors. All require access to antenatal testing facilities. Recent years have seen a proliferation of maternofetal assessment units or day-care units. The benefits of this include the gathering together of the various tests with the compilation and review of results. Daily outpatient assessment and review may be undertaken where previously admission to hospital was the norm. However, easy access may result in excessive testing with largely normal results. Protocols of referral should be formulated and audit undertaken. An assessment unit should be located near the ultrasound department because testing can be integrated with ultrasound examination. The focus of fetal assessment is the antenatal cardiotocograph (CTG). Appropriate equipment is the Sonicaid Team, Hewlett-Packard 1351, Corometrics 118 or Huntleigh Baby Dopplex 3000. The Sonicaid System 8000 is an additional option which has a particular value in providing electronic storage of the CTG. Caution should be exercised in depending on computerized trace analysis with consequent risk of the loss of human skills of interpretation. A data collection computer has become essential. The unit should be staffed by motivated midwives who can diversify their clinical interest. They should have the support of available and interested medical staff in assessment of problem cases. The individual requesting the test should be aware of the result in order to plan and justify the further management. This should not be delegated by default to a junior member of staff.

IDENTIFICATION OF THE FETUS AT RISK

There are two groups of women who may require fetal assessment:

1. Women with previously recognized historical risk factors such as previous stillbirth and neonatal death, or medical disorders such as diabetes mellitus, hypertension or other conditions.
2. Lower-risk women who develop obstetric complications during pregnancy such as antepartum haemorrhage, hypertension, reduced fetal movement, intrauterine growth restriction, cholestasis or prolongation of pregnancy.

Adverse outcome due to prematurity or acute events like cord occlusion or placental abruption cannot be predicted by existing tests of fetal wellbeing. Fetal testing on account of the above markers within the past history can only be for maternal reassurance and should be minimized; excessive testing may generate anxiety *and consume much needed resources.* Chronic compromise due to placental insufficiency operates through growth or nutritional failure of varying degrees. Some of these adverse results might be prevented by identification of the fetus at risk and appropriate intervention. Hypoxia is not the only mechanism of compromise; other conditions like diabetes mellitus, Rhesus isoimmunization and maternal or fetal infection may present a different threat. Selection of tests appropriate to the condition is important. There should be a protocol for testing which is related to the condition.

Cases are referred for fetal assessment for a variety of reasons. The most common indications are an abdominal size inappropriate for gestational age and reduced fetal movements. Vaginal bleeding, premature labour, prolongation of pregnancy and hypertension are also common.

FETAL GROWTH

The abdomen may be judged to be a different size from that expected from the dates. More commonly this is smaller rather than larger. The importance of detecting small babies in utero has been emphasized in Chapter 2.

The use of the term 'intrauterine growth retardation' has led to much confusion with disagreement on how it should be defined. The word 'restriction' should replace the word 'retardation' because of the possibility of misunderstanding of the meaning of this word by the mother.

The clinical scenario may indicate a risk of hypoxic intrauterine growth restriction (IUGR) in well-recognized situations: previous IUGR baby, malnourished mother, smoking, alcohol, drug abuse, medical conditions, gestational hypertension, multiple pregnancy and other conditions. The measurement of the fundosymphysis height (see Figs 2.1 and 2.2) in cm, given that the fetus is a single fetus in a longitudinal lie, is plotted on a chart or simply compared with the gestational age in weeks. If it is more than 2 cm smaller than the gestational age before 36 weeks or 3 cm thereafter, then it is clinically small for dates. The confounding effects of abnormal lie, obesity, fibroids, multiple pregnancy and polyhydramnios have already been mentioned.

Clinically small for dates is an indication for an ultrasound scan.

On ultrasound examination measurements of head circumference (HC), abdominal circumference (AC) and femur length (FL) are taken and plotted on a growth chart (Fig. 6.1). The AC reflects fetal weight most accurately and if it falls below the 5th centile, this is ultrasonically small for dates. Customized fundosymphysial growth charts based on ethnicity, parity, height and weight of the mother are available (www.gestation.net)[19] and are said to identify more cases of

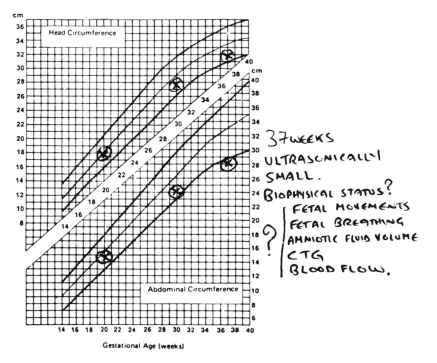

Figure 6.1 Ultrasound chart: small for dates

IUGR than conventional measurement with the tape which is plotted on a 'gravidogram' (fundosymphysial height plotted in relation to gestation). Similarly customized growth charts are available to plot the estimated fetal weight based on ultrasound measurements.[19] A fetus that is ultrasonically small may be an expected small baby due to small parents, i.e. genetic smallness. Alternatively a small fetus may be pathologically small due to an abnormal process. To distinguish one from the other the following should be taken into account:

- risk factors
- amniotic fluid volume
- subjective and objective fetal movements
- CTG
- other biophysical elements: fetal breathing, fetal tone, blood flow velocity waveform in the fetal vessels by Doppler ultrasound.

Pathological smallness is what is generally referred to as intrauterine growth restriction. This term carries an implication of a likelihood of a hypoxic process being present. The pathology of growth restriction is defined by the size but function is more important.

Not all small fetuses are suffering from IUGR.

A growth-restricted baby is one that has not realized its own intrinsic growth potential.

The growth-restricted baby identified before or on admission in labour is flagged for special care with continuous electronic fetal monitoring, careful use of oxytocic therapy when needed and no undue prolongation of the labour process. The final proof of hypoxic IUGR comes from the neonatologist's observations of weight (in relation to expected weight for gestational age) and neonatal behaviour. Usually these babies have a scaphoid abdomen, little subcutaneous fat deposition in the limbs and can be recognized by measurement of ponderal indices.

BIOPHYSICAL MONITORING OF FETAL HEALTH

Fetal movements

Fetal activity in the form of fetal movement perceived by the mother is a reliable indicator of fetal health. Women should be encouraged to be aware of this. A reduction in fetal movement of concern to the mother is an indication for careful assessment, initially by CTG followed by an ultrasound assessment. An appropriate abdominal circumference and normal amniotic fluid volume on ultrasound are reassuring and often the fetus is seen to be active during the scan. The woman will also see this and be reassured. Commonly the fetus recommences normal movements and there is no need for further assessment.

In a randomized study involving 68 000 women routine use of fetal movement charts was not beneficial compared with more selective use.[20] Reduced or no movements predicted poor perinatal outcome but this could not be prevented. This may be partly to do with different reporting times in the study and inadequate surveillance, i.e. late surveillance or being only dependent on the CTG. The commonly-used chart is the Cardiff 'Count to Ten' chart. Sadovsky, who studied fetal movement extensively, suggested that there should be four fetal movements in a 30-min period during one day of which one has to be strong.[21] The expectation of four fetal movements in 30 min or 10 in 12 h is arbitrary and correlated with good perinatal outcome.[22-24] A single fetal movement felt by the mother may not be recorded by the ultrasound movement detection devices. However, when a mother feels clusters of fetal movements for 15–20 s it is detected by the ultrasound transducer and is almost always associated with fetal heart rate (FHR) accelerations (see Fig. 5.19).[25] Women should be encouraged to be reassured by clusters of fetal movements.

The commonest answer to the question 'Is the baby moving?' is 'Yes, a lot'. We have to be prepared for the next question 'Can it move too much? Can this be bad?' There are many anecdotal reports by experienced clinicians of excessive fetal movements followed by death in utero. This must be due to an acute event and cord accidents or abruption could be postulated. In-utero convulsions do occur whether due to pre-existing brain abnormality or another mechanism and may be reported by the mother as excessive fetal movement followed by death. In any event it must be extremely rare and this should not compromise our general reassurance of the mother that a lot of fetal movement is a healthy phenomenon. When a woman complains of excessive fetal movements a reversion to normal movements is reassuring but if there is subsequent absent fetal movements she should attend urgently for review.

Increased fetal activity can lead to confluence of accelerations mimicking a fetal tachycardia, and the synchronous automatic recording of fetal movements as done by the newest monitors will help to clarify this situation.[26] There are monitors using actograms that attempt to record fetal movement and fetal breathing in addition to the FHR. The clinical application of this principle remains to be proven.

Antepartum electronic fetal heart rate monitoring

Non-stress test

The recording of the FHR for a period of 20–30 min without any induced stress to the fetus (like oxytocin infusion or nipple stimulation) to produce uterine contractions is called the non-stress test (NST). In the UK this is commonly referred to as an antenatal CTG. The duration of this test should be until reactivity is observed; until there are two accelerations in a 10-min period. The sleep phase with no fetal movement and no FHR accelerations does not exceed 40 min in the vast majority of healthy fetuses and almost all healthy fetuses show a reactive trace within 90 min.[27] This forms the framework for extending the NST for 40 min when it is not reactive in the first 20 min. In some centres vibro-acoustic stimulus is used to provoke activity if there is no reactivity for 40 min.

A summary of the interpretation of the NST based on the International Federation of Obstetrics and Gynaecology (FIGO) recommendations[12] and the actions that are recommended with each type of trace are given below.

Antepartum cardiotocograph (NST)

Normal/reassuring

- At least two accelerations (>15 beats for >15 s) in 10 min (reactive trace), baseline heart rate 110–150 beats per min (bpm), baseline variability 5–25 bpm, absence of decelerations.
- Sporadic mild decelerations (amplitude <40 bpm, duration <30 s) are acceptable following an acceleration.
- When there is moderate tachycardia (150–170 bpm) or bradycardia (100–110 bpm), a reactive trace without decelerations is reassuring of good health.

Interpretation/action: Repeat according to clinical situation and the degree of fetal risk.

Suspicious/equivocal

- Absence of accelerations for >40 min (non-reactive).
- Baseline heart rate 150–170 bpm or 110–100 bpm, baseline variability >25 bpm in the absence of accelerations.
- Sporadic decelerations of any type unless severe as described below.

Interpretation/action: Continue for 90 min until trace becomes reactive, or repeat CTG within 24 h, or vibro-acoustic stimulation (VAS)/

amniotic fluid index (AFI)/biophysical profile (BPP)/Doppler ultrasound blood velocity waveform.

Pathological/abnormal

- Baseline heart rate <100 bpm or >170 bpm.
- Silent pattern <5 bpm for >90 min.
- Sinusoidal pattern (oscillation frequency <2–5 cycles/min, amplitude of 2–10 bpm for >40 min with no acceleration and no area of normal baseline variability).
- Repeated late, prolonged (>1 min) and severe variable (>40 bpm) decelerations.

Interpretation/action: Further evaluation (VAS, AFI, BPP, Doppler ultrasound blood velocity waveform). Deliver if clinically appropriate.

The antepartum cardiotocograph (NST) is usually applied for diagnostic purposes; its value for screening has not been proven.[12] Pooled results of four studies of NSTs involving 10 169 patients revealed a satisfactory outcome with a false negative rate of 7 per 10 000 cases.[28–31] In order to reduce the number of non-reactive NSTs fetal VAS to produce FHR accelerations has been employed.[32] The perinatal outcome based on the results of the FHR tracing obtained after VAS has been shown to be as reliable as the results of the NST without VAS.[33]

The NST may be abnormal not only due to hypoxia but due to other causes associated with reduced baseline variability as discussed in Chapter 5. A review of the history with further evaluation will be helpful to clarify the cause.

Contraction stress test (CST)/oxytocin challenge test (OCT)

When the NST is not reactive for 40 min or longer, it has been the practice in some centres to perform an OCT. It is carried out using intravenous oxytocin infusion starting with 2.5 mU/min and increasing by 2.5 mU/min every 20–30 min until three contractions are observed over 10 min. In cases of women with a previous uterine scar, oxytocin can be started at 1.0 mU/min and increased by 1.0 mU/min every 20–30 min. Absence of either decelerations or accelerations, or isolated decelerations, make the test inconclusive. Repeated late or variable decelerations with at least half the induced uterine contractions indicate a fetus that may become compromised antenatally or in labour. Two accelerations in a 10-min period and absence of decelerations despite contractions indicate a healthy fetus.

Comparative studies have shown fetal acoustic stimulation (FAST) used to elicit accelerations in a non-reactive trace has a similar predictive value as a contraction stress test.[34] Compared to OCT, a VAS test is easier, cheaper, quicker and can be carried out in an outpatient clinic. It is also safer than OCT in patients with an over-distended uterus, with uterine scar and in the preterm period. Depending on the availability of other methods of testing of a biophysical nature, there is probably no place for OCT in current obstetric practice.

Assessment of amniotic fluid volume

Fetal urine contributes significantly to amniotic fluid volume. Fetuses with no kidneys have severe oligohydramnios. With diminished placental function and reduced renal perfusion the amniotic fluid volume decreases. Perinatal outcome is poor when the amniotic fluid volume is reduced at delivery.[35,36]

Clinical evaluation by abdominal palpation can be deceptive. The impression of the amniotic fluid volume gained on ultrasound examination is fairly reliable. Objective assessment of the vertical depth of the largest pocket of amniotic fluid after excluding loops of cord or the sum of the vertical pockets in the four quadrants of the uterus (amniotic fluid index (AFI)) is used in practice. AFI correlates well with changes in amniotic fluid volume during the course of pregnancy[37,38] and there is little inter- or intraobserver variation.[39,40] The AFI is more sensitive in predicting fetal morbidity than the largest single vertical pocket of amniotic fluid.[41] An amniotic fluid index of <5 cm is associated with poor fetal outcome[42] and delivery should be considered, assuming reasonable gestational age. If only one vertical pocket is measured, a value of <3 cm in the largest pool is an indication for delivery.

In post-term pregnancy or that complicated by severe growth restriction, the decline in fluid volume can be up to one third every week, and twice-weekly assessment is advisable. Combining AFI and NST with FAST when necessary to provoke accelerations is one of the commonest first-line assessments in high-risk pregnancies and is adequate for most women.[33] No unexpected fetal deaths occurred within one week of performing the test (AFI and NST with FAST) in a series of 6000 cases.[43] Antepartum fetal death within a week of a reactive NST may occur for those who have an AFI below 5.[44] It is quite possible for a fetus with a reactive NST and good fetal movements to die suddenly in the presence of marked oligohydramnios (Fig. 6.2A–C). This may be due to umbilical cord compression. Most centres now recognize that for high-risk pregnancies where a reduction of amniotic fluid volume is suspected (e.g. IUGR, post-term, etc.), it is desirable to perform an AFI. A schematic diagram incorporating AFI and NST with FAST as the first-line assessment is shown in Figure 6.3.

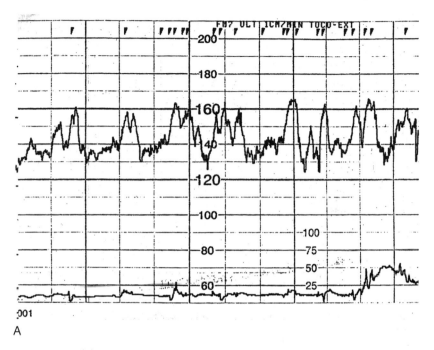

A

Figure 6.2 (A) NST in a post-mature fetus: variability and fetal movements seen

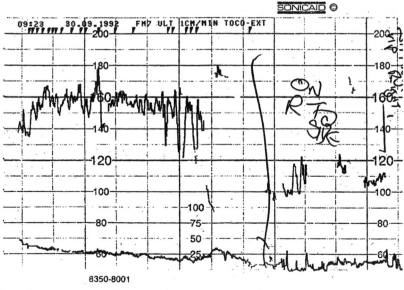

B

Figure 6.2 (B) Sudden decelerations

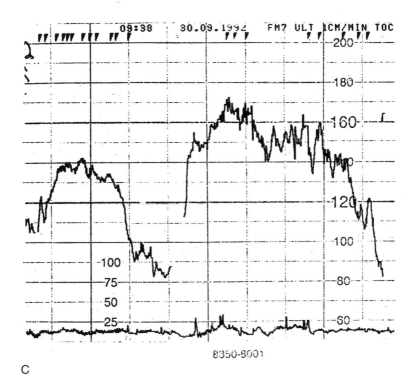

C

Figure 6.2 (C) Bradycardia and fetal death within minutes

Measurement of blood flow velocity waveforms

Sometimes it is not possible to deliver a fetus at risk of progressive hypoxia because of prematurity. There is difficulty in interpreting the NST at early gestations. Measurement of blood flow velocity waveforms in the umbilical artery, fetal aorta and middle cerebral artery may give additional useful information for the timing of delivery in these circumstances.

Biophysical profile

Fetal responses to hypoxia do not occur at random but are initiated and regulated by complex, integrated reflexes of the fetal central nervous system. Stimuli that regulate the biophysical characteristics of fetal movement, breathing and tone arise from different sites in the brain. There is some evidence that the first physical activity to develop is fetal tone at 8 weeks' gestation. It is also the last to cease

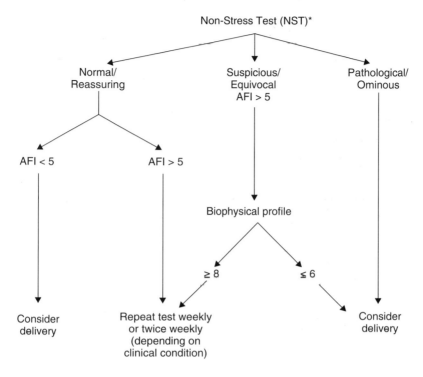

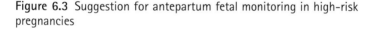

AFI–Amniotic fluid index
*Repeat NST and AFI weekly or more often acording to clinical situation.
In preterm situations additional tests (e.g. Doppler velocimetry) may be of value

Figure 6.3 Suggestion for antepartum fetal monitoring in high-risk pregnancies

functioning when subjected to increasing hypoxia.[45] Fetal movements develop at 9 weeks and fetal breathing at 20 weeks. FHR activity matures last by about 28 weeks and is the first to be affected by hypoxia. In hypoxia, FHR characteristics may become abnormal first followed by breathing, body and limb movements, and finally by tone.

Evaluation of more than one biophysical parameter to assess fetal health has been suggested but it may not be necessary if the NST is reactive and AFI is normal. In the assessment of biophysical profile fetal movements, tone, breathing and amniotic fluid volume assessed by the scan and NST are considered, and for each a score of 2 or 0 is given, there being no intermediate score.[46] When the NST is not reactive, as is more common in the preterm period, it might be useful to assess the fetal biophysical profile. A score of 8 or 10 indicates a fetus in good condition. Retesting should be performed at intervals depending on the level of risk. In situations where the compromise may develop faster, as in prolonged pregnancy, IUGR and prelabour rupture of membranes, it is best performed twice weekly. If the score is 6, then the score should be re-evaluated 4–6 h later and a decision made based on the new score. When the biophysical profile is ≤2 on one occasion, or ≤4 on two occasions (6–8 h apart), delivery of the fetus is indicated if the fetus is adequately mature and has a good chance of survival.[47] Further evaluation with fetal blood flow velocity waveform measurement may be considered if the fetus is so premature that deferring delivery even by a few days is considered beneficial. Good perinatal outcome has been reported with biophysical profile scoring in high-risk pregnancy[47] and as a primary modality of testing in prolonged pregnancy.[48]

A modified biophysical profile where only the ultrasound parameters are evaluated (without NST) has been found to be equally reliable.[49] Due to the time and expertise needed to perform a biophysical profile, many centres perform an NST (if necessary with FAST when NST is not reactive) and an AFI.

Fetal actogram

Three of the five features of a biophysical profile, fetal heart rate pattern, movement and breathing, can be assessed by use of an actogram. An actogram is a recording that can be obtained by a modified FHR monitor which will record the fetal breathing and body movements in addition to the FHR and uterine contractions[50] (Fig. 6.4). Such equipment is used in some centres. If it is found to be reliable, 'biophysical profile' testing would be easier adding more information to the NST. With increasing hypoxia (as in IUGR) or when infection supervenes, the fetus tends to reduce its fetal body and limb movements and its breathing movements. An actogram or biophysical profile done on a daily basis or every other day could suggest an increasing threat. The actocardiograph monitor is less expensive and the recording can be done with ease by a trained paramedical person, compared with the expensive technology and expertise needed to perform a biophysical profile. This approach might be attractive except for the absence of an amniotic fluid volume assessment.

Assessment of the fetus in an outpatient clinic with limited facilities

With gradually increasing hypoxia, FHR changes take place first, followed by alterations in breathing movements, body movements and, finally, the tone. However, sudden demise can occur despite a normal FHR pattern when there is reduced amniotic fluid.[44] When

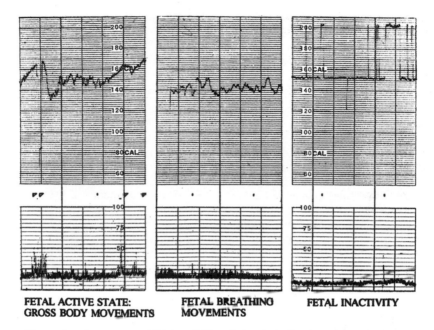

FETAL ACTIVE STATE: GROSS BODY MOVEMENTS   **FETAL BREATHING MOVEMENTS**   **FETAL INACTIVITY**

Figure 6.4 Actogram exhibiting FHR and signals indicative of fetal body and breathing movements

there is fetal body movement for over 3 s it is associated with FHR accelerations.[51] The clinical outcome is similar when the NST is reactive with or without FAST to produce accelerations.[33] It is therefore possible to simplify fetal assessment at the outpatient clinic. A handheld Doptone with a digital display will give a baseline FHR, and application of FAST at this time will result in maternal and observer perception of fetal movement and FHR acceleration, which will be displayed by the doptone.[52] If the fetus continues to move, there will be further accelerations; and in a biophysical profile scoring, these two features (FHR accelerations and fetal movement) will indicate a score of 4. Since tone is the last feature to disappear it is fair to give 2 points for tone when the fetal movements are plentiful with FHR accelerations observed on the Doptone. Low-cost printers are being developed which, when connected to a Doptone, can print a FHR trace similar to that obtained from a conventional CTG monitor (Fig. 6.5). This enables the midwife to perform an NST in the home environment without difficulty.

NST is usually used for diagnostic purposes and has not been proven to be of value as a screening test. The ability of the test to identify the problem being investigated should be known. A normal

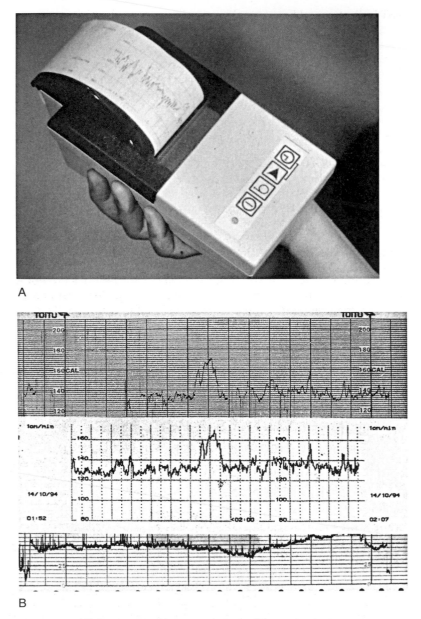

Figure 6.5 (A) Doptone and low-cost printer; (B) an identical trace with a conventional fetal monitor

NST indicates fetal health/wellbeing. However, with chronic placental dysfunction, fetal adaptation occurs and normal (reactive) NST does not indicate the degree by which placental function may be reduced. Thus, the predictive value of a normal NST is governed by the clinical situation.

CASE ILLUSTRATIONS

The NST may not be normal due to a variety of causes other than hypoxia: cardiac arrhythmias, brain abnormality (congenital or acquired), chromosomal abnormality, anaesthesia, drug effects and infection.

Hypoxia

Severe IUGR is seen in the preterm period. It has been suggested that decelerations are a normal feature of the preterm CTG. There is a reduction in variability, and lower amplitude accelerations are seen in the preterm CTG (Fig. 6.6), however major decelerations are not a normal feature. In the preterm period short sharp decelerations of <15 secs may be seen. They are often seen with change of sleep to wake state and may follow immediately after the acceleration. When major decelerations occur the clinical situation should be considered. Figure 6.7 is from a known case of severe IUGR at 25 weeks' gestation. There was oligohydramnios, poor fetal movement and very abnormal fetal and maternal blood flow. On account of a very small fetal weight estimate and early gestation, the couple, with the advice

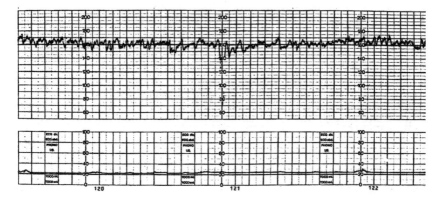

Figure 6.6 CTG in preterm baby: low amplitude accelerations and short sharp decelerations

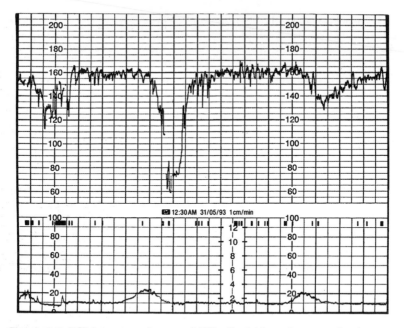

Figure 6.7 NST in a case of severe IUGR, oligohydramnios, poor fetal movement and abnormal fetal and poor maternal blood flow

of the obstetrician, opted for conservative management. The fetus died in utero 3 days later.

Given a bigger weight estimate and later gestation, delivery would have been appropriate. There will be no guarantee that the baby is not already damaged, however there is a good chance such a baby will do well with good neonatal intensive care.[53] Leaving a fetus to die in utero is difficult in the face of reasonable weight and gestation.

Cardiac arrhythmias

Fetal arrhythmia may give rise to an abnormal trace, although the fetus is not hypoxic. Figure 6.8A was obtained from a case where the midwife auscultated the fetal heart in the antenatal clinic and heard a tachycardia. She noted that the multiparous woman was classically low risk and that the fetus was well grown and moving. This was confirmed by ultrasound scan after referral to hospital. Twenty hours later the CTG was repeated and was essentially unchanged. Advice was sought from a specialized unit, a diagnosis of fetal supraventricular tachycardia was made and the administration of double the adult dose of digoxin was recommended. Fetal echocardiography was normal. Figure 6.8B was recorded the following day. The preg-

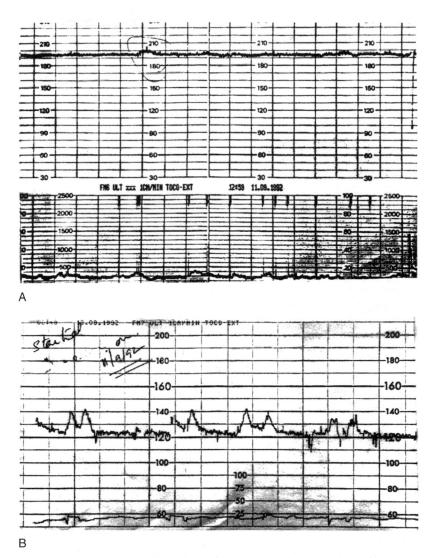

A

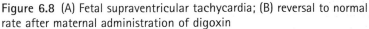

B

Figure 6.8 (A) Fetal supraventricular tachycardia; (B) reversal to normal rate after maternal administration of digoxin

nancy continued, culminating in normal labour, normal intrapartum CTG and normal delivery of a healthy baby two weeks later. The baby had a structurally normal heart and no further problem with the heart rhythm. Figure 6.9 is a similar case but the observation of supraventricular tachycardia was made in early labour. Advice was sought and the administration of digoxin considered inappropriate

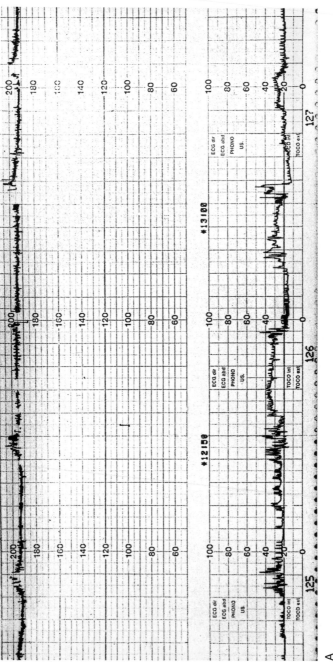

A

Figure 6.9 (A) Supraventricular tachycardia diagnosed in labour

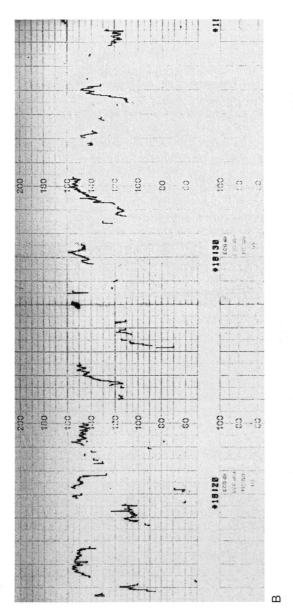

B

Figure 6.9 (*continued*) (B) reversal to normal heart rate with decelerations in the second stage of labour

because the drug would not have taken effect until after the baby had been born. The baby was noted to be moving and continued to do so during labour. The amniotic fluid was clear and the woman was low risk. The CTG remained unchanged during the 6 h of labour until the second stage. At this time the features changed, possibly due to vagal stimulation with descent of the head. Although technically imperfect there appeared to be a normal rate, variability and second stage decelerations (Fig. 6.9B). After delivery the baby had a normal heart rate and no further problem!

Heart block

This can be complete or partial, continuous or intermittent. Occasional dropped beats are frequent and of no significance: they generally do not interfere with the appearance of the trace or persist after delivery. A case of maternal systemic lupus erythematosus with fetal heart block has been shown in Figure 5.24.

Brain abnormalities – acquired

Physiological mechanisms controlling the fetal heart require the integrity of the central nervous system.

An abnormal CTG with no accelerations or decelerations and markedly reduced baseline variability was recorded (Fig. 6.10A) when a high-risk woman on antihypertensive medication presented with a sudden cessation of fetal movement. The fetus was well grown and the amniotic fluid volume was normal on ultrasound scan. During a prolonged scan the fetus did not move. There was a collapsed stomach and an atonic dilated bladder with evidence of a large cerebral haemorrhage (Fig. 6.10B). In view of the unusual findings a fetal blood sample was obtained from the umbilical vein for karyotyping, fetal haematology and cytomegalovirus screening. The fetal blood gases were normal and the fetal haemoglobin was 8 g/dl (1.24 mmol/l) consistent with the intracranial haemorrhage. While the karyotype results were awaited the fetus did not move and died 24 h after the procedure. Post mortem confirmed the cerebral haemorrhage. This severely 'brain-damaged' fetus was not hypoxic and, if delivered, would have had a very poor prognosis. The mother accepted and understood the outcome: she has since had a living child. Intracranial haemorrhage may occur in cases of alloimmune thrombocytopenia or when the woman is on warfarin therapy. When a CTG becomes abnormal despite good growth and good amniotic fluid volume such unusual causes must be considered before deciding to deliver. Delivery will not lead to an improved outcome in these circumstances. In twin-to-twin transfusion syndrome when one fetus dies, the 'second fetus' may suffer from the consequences of sudden haemodynamic changes which may affect the brain and then manifest as a non-reactive CTG. No changes in blood gases on fetal blood sampling or obvious ultrasonic morphological change in the brain are seen immediately but vacuolation in the brain may follow.

Brain abnormalities – congenital

The inability to maintain a steady baseline heart rate (Fig. 6.11A) can be due to severe hypoxic brain damage or may be associated with severe brain malformation. If the fetus is active, indicated by fetal movements, it is unlikely to be hypoxic and the cause of such a trace should be sought by further investigation. The associated pathology in Figure 6.11 was holoprosencephaly shown by ultrasound examination (Fig. 6.11B).

Chromosomal abnormality

A 39-year-old multiparous woman was referred from another hospital with a well-grown fetus, reduced fetal movements and a good volume of amniotic fluid, and yet an abnormal CTG (Fig. 6.12). The Doppler blood flow studies in fetus and mother were normal. There was a slightly reduced femur length and slight hydronephrosis. Delivery was deferred until the result of karyotype from a fetal blood

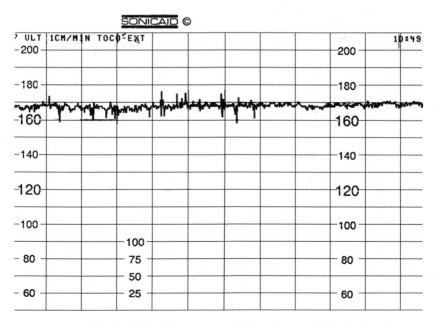

Figure 6.10 (A) CTG with a 'silent pattern' (baseline variability <5 bpm), no accelerations or decelerations

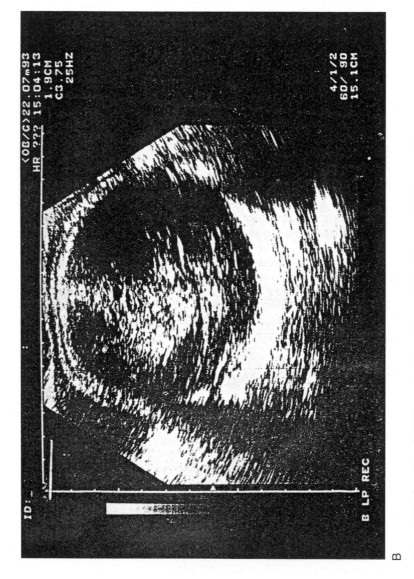

B

Figure 6.10 *(continued)* (B) Scan showing evidence of fetal intracerebral haemorrhage

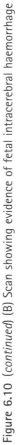

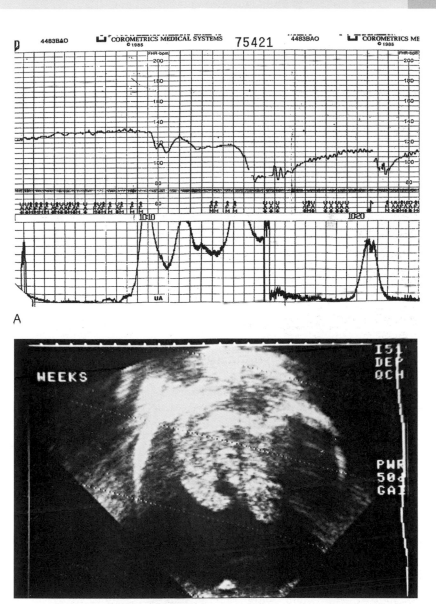

A

B

Figure 6.11 (A) CTG: unsteady baseline but with plenty of fetal movement;
(B) scan showing the fetus with holoprosencephaly

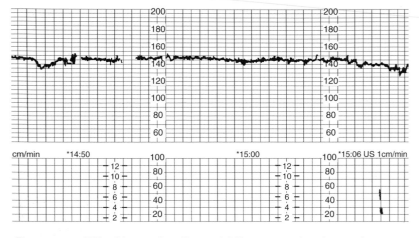

Figure 6.12 CTG with poor baseline variability, no accelerations and isolated decelerations. Misfit of fetal wellbeing tests; abnormal karyotype

sample was known. The fetus died in utero the day before the result, showing Down's syndrome, became available. The mother had been counselled of this strong possibility and requested the baby not to be delivered without the karyotype result.

In chromosomally abnormal fetuses, especially trisomies, the central neural pathway may be disorganized resulting in an abnormal CTG,[54] although the fetal growth, amniotic fluid volume and fetal movements may be normal. In trisomy 13 and 18 the fetus might be growth restricted with an increased amniotic fluid volume. In a proportion of these cases the CTG shows a steady baseline but with poor baseline variability, reduced or absent accelerations and isolated decelerations. The disorganized neural development may manifest after birth as mental retardation.

A misfit of fetal function tests suggests the need for further investigations.

Fetal anaemia

This may show a sinusoidal or sinusoidal-like pattern and is discussed in Chapter 10.

Anaesthesia

The fetus is anaesthetized as well as the mother! The fetus may excrete the drugs more slowly than the mother. A multiparous woman fractured her tibia at 29 weeks' gestation. She was given a general anaesthetic in order to insert a pin and plate. A CTG performed on her return from the operating theatre 2 h after induction of anaesthesia showed a dramatic reduction of baseline variability and the absence of accelerations (Fig. 6.13A). The inexperienced junior doctor suspected hypoxia and thought delivery might be necessary. Ultrasound scan confirmed a well-grown fetus and reasonable amniotic fluid volume. The consultant recommended a repeat CTG 2 h later (Fig. 6.13B) and another 24 h after that (Fig. 6.13C). The pregnancy progressed normally to term without further complication.

Drug effects

Sedatives, tranquillizers, antihypertensives and other drugs which act on the central nervous system tend to reduce the amplitude of the accelerations and suppress the baseline variability. In these situations other forms of surveillance become necessary. With antihypertensive therapy fetal activity may be unaffected.

Infections

A fetal tachycardia associated with a maternal infection is a cause for concern. The mechanism may be direct fetal infection or secondary response of the fetus due to transplacental passage of pyrogens or adrenergic metabolites. When fetal tachycardia occurs with maternal tachycardia due to maternal urinary tract infection it usually settles with antibiotic treatment. However, when fetal tachycardia persists for a considerable period of time then the fetus may not be able to tolerate it. Consideration of the clinical picture will suggest whether an actual fetal infection is likely. Preservation of baseline variability and reactivity suggests a resilient fetus.

If there is reduced variability with or without decelerations in the absence of accelerations, the fetus itself is sick. A mother was admitted with a systemic illness at 33 weeks' gestation and tachycardia. On assumption of the diagnosis of urinary tract infection a cephalosporin was prescribed. The trace showed tachycardia with markedly reduced variability and shallow decelerations (Fig. 6.14). The mother's condition did not improve nor did the fetal heart tracing. Rupture of the membranes with the release of meconium-stained amniotic fluid prompted caesarean section. The baby succumbed within hours of birth to congenital listeriosis; it was heavily infected. This is reflected in the seriously abnormal fetal heart tracing.

Maternal illness and preterm meconium suggest possible listerial infection.

Suspicion of the diagnosis, blood cultures and treatment with ampicillin might have led to a better outcome.[55]

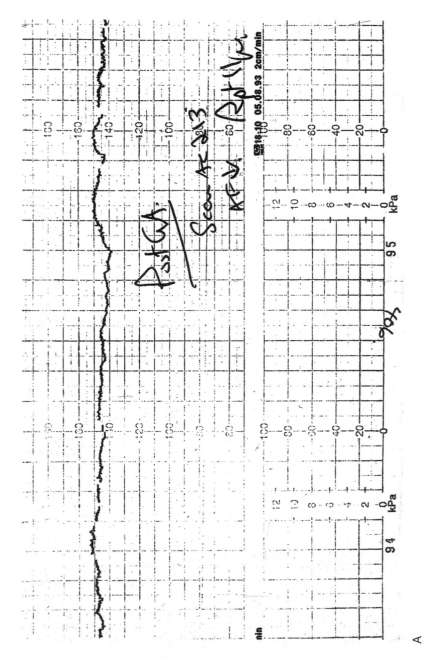

Figure 6.13 (A) CTG performed 2 h after induction of anaesthesia: no accelerations and reduced baseline variability

A

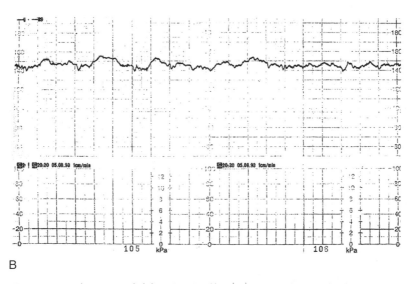

B

Figure 6.13 (*continued*) (B) CTG 4 h after induction of anaesthesia

In cases with prelabour rupture of the membranes a CTG showing tachycardia, lack of accelerations and reduced variability suggests a higher probability of infection even in the absence of clinical signs.

REDUCED FETAL MOVEMENTS

This is a frequent reason for fetal assessment. A CTG on its own should not be taken as providing full reassurance in this situation. Even if the CTG is normal at the time of recording there might subsequently have been decelerations due to cord compression and oligohydramnios. Reassurance can only be obtained on this issue by finding a normal AFI of more than 8. A value of 5–8 is reduced and the test should be repeated depending on the clinical situation: generally in 3–4 days. If the fetal growth is satisfactory, AFI is normal and CTG is satisfactory no further assessment is immediately indicated. In such cases the movements frequently resume, often during the testing!

PROLONGED PREGNANCY

This is a common indication for assessment in many hospitals. The clinician will have reviewed the menstrual and ultrasound dating and most cases will have reached 41 weeks. The CTG may be normal but caution should be applied in being reassured by this. Figure 6.2

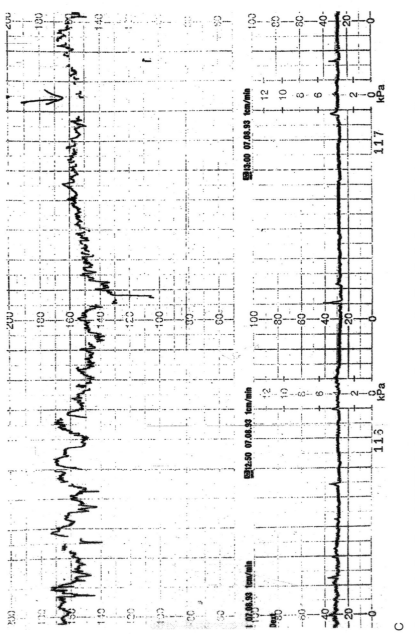

C

Figure 6.13 (continued) (C) CTG 24 h later – reactive trace after the effect of anaesthesia has worn off

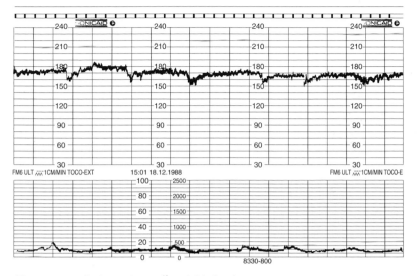

Figure 6.14 Ominous trace: listerial infection

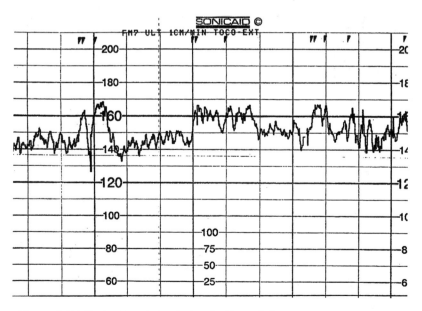

Figure 6.15 Postmature intrauterine death next day

was obtained in the assessment unit in a case where the maturity was 42 weeks and 5 days. Two days previously the deepest pool of amniotic fluid had been 3.2 cm and the CTG was reactive. On the day of assessment the CTG was the first investigation to be performed. Fetal movements are seen on the trace and the first 7 min suggest reasonable baseline variability although a slightly fast rate. Deep decelerations followed and the woman was transferred to the labour ward. In the anaesthetic room 20 min after the end of the trace, ultrasound scan showed a terminal bradycardia. A decision was made not to deliver and the heart stopped within minutes of observation. The baby was found to be otherwise normal at post-mortem examination. Again the presentation suggests possible cord compression with oligohydramnios as the mechanism. In another case where intrauterine death occurred 24 h after a CTG in a postmature gestation (Fig. 6.15), the CTG had been normal and a single deepest pool of amniotic fluid had been 2 cm. Since that case we have performed AFI measurement during assessment.

AFI should form an integral part of assessment of fetal wellbeing.

Chapter 7

The admission test by cardiotocography or by auscultation

Since the production of the NICE guidelines[13] there has been much discussion about the role of an admission cardiotocograph (CTG). The guidelines suggest that it is not mandatory. This is partly because of the absence of evidence based on randomized controlled trials that it is effective. We hope this chapter will enable caregivers to provide choice to women about this issue.

Fetal morbidity and mortality are greater in high-risk women with hypertension, diabetes, intrauterine growth restriction and other risk factors. A greater number of antenatal deaths are observed in this group. In pregnancies that have proceeded to term, morbidity and mortality due to events in labour occur with similar frequency in those categorized as low risk compared with high risk based on traditional risk classification.[56,57] This may be because high-risk cases such as intrauterine growth restriction have been missed during antenatal care. To resolve this we have to turn our attention to better screening during the antenatal period and at the onset of labour. With traditional assessment the fetal heart is auscultated after admission and every 15 min for a period of 1 min after a contraction in the first stage of labour and every 5 min or after every other contraction in the second stage of labour. During auscultation the baseline fetal heart rate (FHR) can be measured but other features of the FHR such as baseline variability, accelerations and decelerations are more difficult to observe and quantify. Figure 5.28 shows an admission CTG of a fetus in serious trouble with a pathological trace. Auscultation after a contraction by a skilled midwife (indicated by black dots) showed a 'normal' heart rate of 150 beats per min (bpm).

Baseline variability is not audible to the unaided ear.

The features that will provide the reassurance of fetal health are the presence of accelerations, normal baseline variability and an absence of decelerations that outlasts the contractions, i.e. late and atypical variable decelerations.

An admission test (AT) should pick up the apparently low-risk woman whose fetus is compromised on admission or is likely to become compromised in labour. This admission test may be performed by a CTG or by 'intelligent' auscultation.

The AT by CTG is a short, continuous electronic FHR recording made immediately on admission, and gives a better impression of the fetal condition compared with simple auscultation. In many hospitals electronic monitoring is performed but it is done long after admission. The mother may have waited for a bed, a nightdress, general observations to be noted and other administrative issues resolved. In most instances the mother walking into the labour ward is entirely healthy and her main concern is to have a healthy baby. An AT may identify those who are already at risk with an ominous pattern on admission even without any contractions (Fig. 7.1). In those with a normal or suspicious FHR the functional stress of the uterine contractions in early labour may bring about the abnormal FHR changes (Fig. 7.2). These changes may be subtle and difficult to identify by auscultation. Careful review may reveal a reduced FSH and a growth-restricted fetus in such cases. An admission CTG can be considered to function in the same way as a natural oxytocin challenge test.

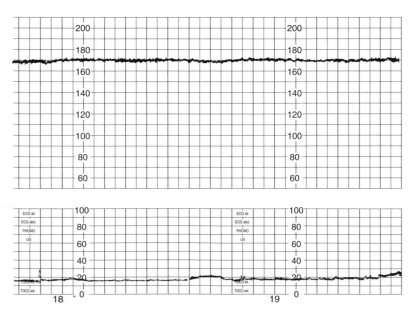

Figure 7.1 Abnormal admission test without contractions

STUDIES ON ADMISSION CARDIOTOCOGRAPHY

In Kandang Kerbau Hospital in Singapore a blinded AT study was carried out on 1041 low-risk women.[58] A FHR tracing was obtained after covering the digital display of the FHR and the recording paper and turning down the volume so that the research midwife had no information about what the FHR trace was showing. The transducer was adjusted based on the green signal light of a fetal monitor (Hewlett-Packard 8040 or 8041) which indicates good signal quality and produces a good tracing. The trace, obtained for 20 min immediately on admission, was sealed in an envelope and put aside for later analysis. These women were a low-risk population based on risk factors and hence were sent to the low-risk labour ward for care by intermittent auscultation. This study was accepted by the departmental ethical committee because the normal practice at that time was that none of the low-risk women had any electronic monitoring.

For this study a reactive normal FHR trace was defined as a recording with normal baseline rate and variability, two accelerations of 15 beats above the baseline for 15 s, and no decelerations. A 'suspicious' or 'equivocal' trace was one that had no accelerations in addition to one abnormal feature such as reduced baseline variability (<5 bpm), presence of decelerations, baseline tachycardia or bradycardia. A trace was classified as 'ominous' when more than one abnormal feature or repeated atypical variable or late decelerations were present. To evaluate the outcome, 'fetal distress' was considered to be present when ominous FHR changes led to caesarean

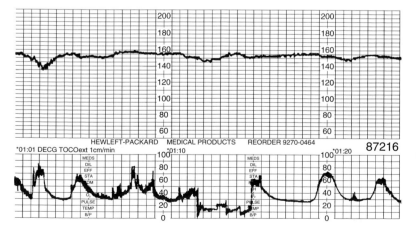

Figure 7.2 Contraction stress is often present in an admission test

section or forceps delivery, or if the newborn had an Apgar score <7 at 5 min after spontaneous delivery (Table 7.1).

In women with ominous ATs (n = 10), 40% developed fetal distress compared with 1.4% (13 out of 982) in those with a reactive AT. Of those 13 who developed fetal distress after a reactive AT, 10 did so more than 5 h after the AT. Of the 3 who developed fetal distress in less than 5 h, one had cord prolapse (baby born by caesarean section in good condition) and the other 2 fetuses were less than 35 weeks' gestation. They had low Apgar scores at birth 3 and 4 h after the AT but needed minimal resuscitation. In those with an ominous AT there was 1 fresh stillbirth of a normally-formed baby with normal birth weight for gestational age at term. The midwife was charting the FHR as 140/min every 20 min for 2 h when she reported that she was unable to hear the FHR. The admission test trace is shown in Figure 7.3. There is no doubt that the midwife's observations were correct; but unfortunately she could not hear the poor baseline variability and

Table 7.1 Results of admission test in relation to the incidence of 'fetal distress'

	Admission test	Fetal distress
REACTIVE	n = 982 (94.3%)	13 (1.4%)
EQUIVOCAL	n = 49 (4.7%)	5 (10.0%)
OMINOUS	n = 10 (1.0%)	4 (40.0%)

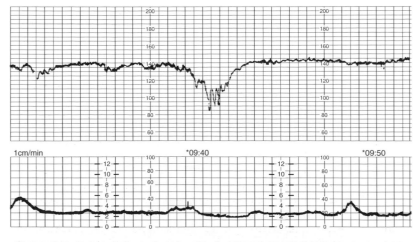

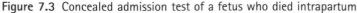

Figure 7.3 Concealed admission test of a fetus who died intrapartum

the shallow decelerations which are ominous features, although the baseline rate was normal.

Barring acute events, the AT may be a good predictor of fetal condition at the time of admission and during the next few hours of labour in term fetuses labelled as low risk. If the AT is normal and reactive, gradually-developing hypoxia will be reflected by no accelerations and by a gradually rising baseline FHR; the latter could be picked up at the time of intermittent auscultation or electronic monitoring. Figure 7.4A–F shows sequential changes in an 8-h labour showing gradual rise of FHR with absent accelerations and reduced baseline variability. Furthermore, it is known that if a well-grown fetus with clear amniotic fluid and a reactive trace starts to develop an abnormal FHR pattern, it takes some time with these FHR changes before acidosis develops. It was estimated that in these situations, for 50% of the babies to become acidotic took 115 min with repeated late decelerations, 145 min with repeated variable decelerations and 185 min with a flat trace.[15] Therefore, it can be safely assumed that if the AT was reactive it is reasonable to perform intermittent auscultation. In some institutions this is further enhanced by 20 min of electronic monitoring 2–3 hourly in low-risk labour.

RANDOMISED CONTROLLED TRIALS ON ADMISSION TEST

A recent systematic review of 3 randomized controlled trials (n = 11 259) and 11 observational studies (n = 5831) suggests that there is no evidence to support the labour admission test.[59] The two large randomized controlled trials[60,61] did not show any benefit in terms of neonatal outcome.

In those who had the admission CTG, the epidural analgesia rate was increased (relative risk (RR) 1.35; 95% confidence interval (CI) 1.1–1.4), as well as the incidence of continuous electronic fetal monitoring (EFM) (RR 1.3; 95% CI 1.2–1.5) and fetal blood sampling (FBS) (RR 1.3; 95% CI 1.1–1.5). The operative delivery rate was the same in the two groups suggesting that this may have been due to the increased fetal scalp blood sampling rate in those who had the admission CTG. The study from Dublin[61] contributed 8580 out of the total of 11 259 cases for this meta-analysis.[59] In the Dublin study[61] the presence of clear amniotic fluid was a prerequisite to enter the study. In order to achieve this, artificial rupture of membranes was performed at a mean cervical dilatation of 1.2 cm. This may not be an acceptable practice in many centres. We believe that the latter study influenced the outcome of the meta-analysis. There were higher rates of continuous EFM and a higher incidence of FBS, and this may be because, in this study, 32% of admission CTGs were considered suspicious or abnormal – an unexpectedly high percentage in early labour in women with clear amniotic fluid. Despite no definitive evidence to

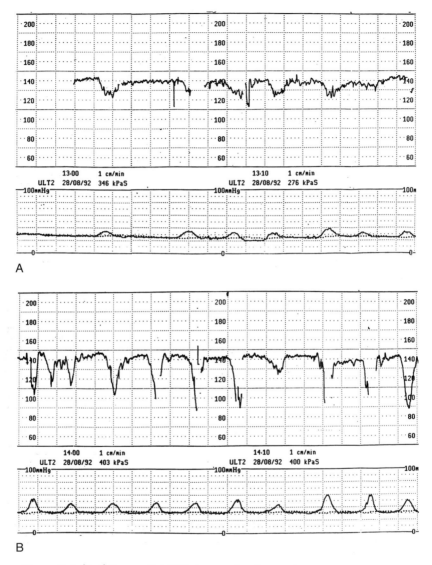

A

B

Figure 7.4 (A–F) Sequential CTG changes to abnormal

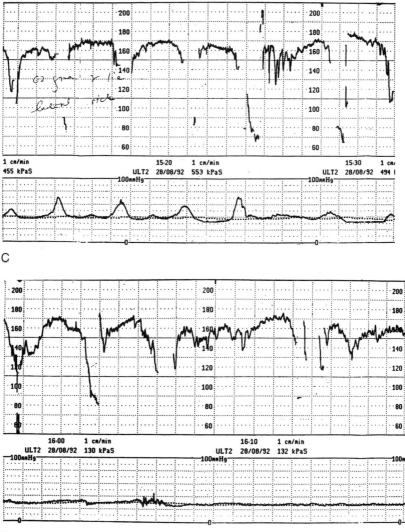

C

D

Figure 7.4 (*continued*)

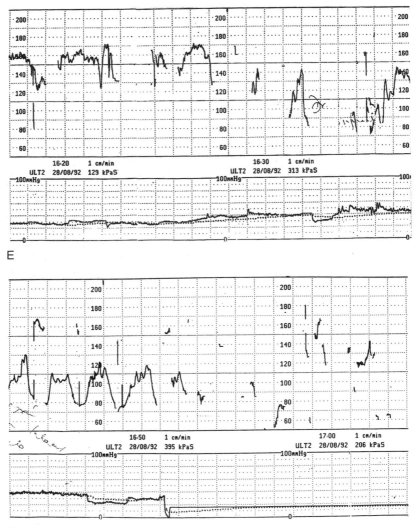

E

F

Figure 7.4 (*continued*)

support admission CTG, it is carried out in many units and the CTG not discontinued, and we believe that this may be due to lack of confidence in interpretation of the CTG or due to the shortage of midwives to provide one-to-one care, including auscultation every 15 min as recommended by NICE.[13]

ADMISSION TEST BY AUSCULTATION ('INTELLIGENT AUSCULTATION')

If we are to limit our practice to auscultation it may be useful to use a Doptone so that the mother and her partner can listen. On admission the mother must be asked the question as to when the baby moved last and the time noted. A baseline FHR can be taken and recorded. With her permission the midwife or doctor could place the hand on the maternal abdomen and ask the mother to notify when she feels the baby moving. The caregiver can note that he/she felt the fetal movements along with the mother, and auscultation at this time should give a heart rate of 15 beats more than the baseline heart rate as accelerations are expected with fetal movements. Continued palpation of the uterus should reveal a contraction, when the FHR should be auscultated. Presence or absence of obvious decelerations should be noted. If fetal movements were felt, the FHR acceleration was heard with the fetal movement, and there was no deceleration with, or soon after, a contraction, then one could reassure the mother of good fetal health. Subsequent observations could be as recommended – to listen every 15 min for 1 min soon after a contraction in the first stage and after every 5 min in the second stage. Non-technological monitoring is undertaken during home births by competent midwives using this principle.

OTHER FORMS OF ADMISSION TEST

The amniotic fluid index (AFI) and Doppler indices of umbilical artery blood flow, to assess fetal wellbeing in early labour, have been evaluated as useful screening tests for fetal distress in labour.[62,63] These tests need expensive equipment and expertise compared with an admission CTG.

Assessment of amniotic fluid volume

Perinatal mortality and morbidity are increased in the presence of reduced amniotic fluid volume at delivery.[35,36] A reproducible semi-quantitative measurement of amniotic fluid volume in early labour could conceivably be used as an adjunct to an admission CTG to triage a fetus to a high- or low-risk status in early labour.[64] In a study involving 120 women in early labour it was found that ultrasound measurement of the vertical depth of two amniotic fluid pockets could be easily and rapidly performed by medical and midwifery staff and that the results were easily reproducible.[65] They found that a vertical depth of two pools of amniotic fluid over 3 cm was highly sensitive and predictive when used as a predictor of the absence of significant fetal distress in the first stage of labour. In this study, 6 women had a vertical depth less than 3 cm; 4 of these women had a caesarean section in the first stage of labour for fetal distress, and in 3 of the newborns the cord pH was <7.2. None of the women who had amniotic fluid volume greater than 3 cm required caesarean section for fetal distress. In a study[66] of 1092 singleton pregnancies, amniotic fluid volume was 'quantified' by measuring the AFI, using the four- quadrant technique.[37] An AFI of less than 5 in early labour, even in the presence of a normal admission CTG, was associated with higher operative delivery rates for fetal distress, low Apgar scores, more infants needing assisted ventilation and a higher admission rate to the neonatal intensive care unit. When the admission CTG was suspicious, an AFI of greater than 5 was associated with better obstetric outcome compared with those with an AFI of less than 5. The low AFI of below 5 may indicate incipient hypoxia and the stress of cord compression, or gradual decline of oxygenation with contractions in labour may be the cause of poor outcome.

Umbilical artery Doppler velocimetry

Umbilical artery Doppler velocimetry has been used as an admission test. It has been shown to be a poor predictor of fetal distress in labour in the low-risk population.[62,67] A larger study of 1092 women has shown Doppler velocimetry on admission to be of little value in the presence of a normal admission CTG. However, in cases with a suspicious admission CTG, normal Doppler velocimetry was associated with less operative deliveries for fetal distress, better Apgar scores and less need for assisted ventilation or admission to the neonatal intensive care unit.[66]

RELATIONSHIP OF NEUROLOGICALLY-IMPAIRED TERM INFANTS TO RESULTS OF ADMISSION TEST

There is controversy regarding the value of continuous EFM let alone an admission test. Other than acute or terminal patterns of prolonged bradycardia or prolonged decelerations of a large amplitude and duration, there is little information regarding FHR patterns and neurological handicap at term[68-71] other than some observation of neurological impairment and non-reactivity,[72-74] especially in the presence of meconium. In an investigation of 48 neurologically-impaired singleton term infants, the admission FHR findings and the FHR patterns 30 min before delivery were analysed.[75] Findings of this investigation are shown in Tables 7.2 and 7.3.

Based on the data in Tables 7.2 and 7.3 it is clear that fetuses with a reactive AT (accelerations) will show the following features prior to or becoming hypoxic: all will exhibit decelerations (100%); almost all will have reduced baseline variability (93%) and tachycardia (93%). The one case where the FHR did not exceed 160 bpm showed an increase in the baseline rate by 25%, and decelerations which can be picked up on auscultation and action taken. On the other hand, if the AT is non-reactive the development of further abnormal features with progress of labour are variable and subtle; this is difficult to recognize by intermittent auscultation. This is because already there might have been hypoxic damage and the fetus is unable to respond. In those with a non-reactive AT nearly 82% had decelerations on the AT and 64% had reduced baseline variability (below 5 bpm) and

Table 7.2 Admission FHR findings in 48 neurologically-impaired term infants separated on the basis of FHR reactivity

FHR pattern on admission up to 120 min	Reactive (n = 15)	Non-reactive (n = 33)
FHR variability (average)	14 (93%)	12[a] (36%)
Decelerations	2 (13%)	27 (82%)
Tachycardia	0 (0%)	6 (18%)

[a] $P < 0.001$

Table 7.3 FHR pattern in the last 30 min before delivery, separated on the basis of admission fetal heart rate pattern

Admission FHR pattern last 30 minutes before delivery	Reactive (n = 15)	Non-reactive (n = 33)
FHR variability (average)	1 (7%)	11[b] (33%)
Decelerations	15 (100%)	5 (15%)
Tachycardia	14[a] (93%)	9[c] (27%)

[a] The baseline FHR in one case did not rise >160 bpm to be defined as tachycardia but showed an increase in baseline FHR of 25%.[75]
[b] $P < 0.05$
[c] $P < 0.001$

many (82%) had a normal baseline rate. The fact that a hypoxic fetus can have a normal baseline rate and shallow decelerations of less than 15 bpm in a non-reactive trace when the baseline variability is below 5 bpm is not widely known (see Fig. 7.3).

All fetuses who exhibited a reactive AT had decelerations and a gradually increasing baseline FHR suggestive of developing fetal hypoxia. It is not difficult to identify this increase in baseline FHR on auscultation (see Fig. 11.13a–j). A recent randomized study compared the obstetric outcome in a group who had intermittent auscultation and 2-hourly 20 min of CTG following the admission test with a group who had continuous EFM.[76] The obstetric outcome, in terms of operative delivery, low Apgar scores and admission to the neonatal unit, was the same in the two groups. The interval between admission to the labour ward to first detected FHR abnormality was the same in the two groups. This finding reassures that FHR can be confidently auscultated for changes that will indicate 'fetal distress' if the AT showed a reactive trace. On the other hand, if the trace was non-reactive with silent pattern (baseline variability below 5) for over 90 min with shallow or no decelerations, the fetus may already be compromised or is likely to be compromised. Action should be taken to establish the acid–base status by FBS or delivery should be considered. Failure to take action may end in fetal death (Fig. 7.5a–j). It is

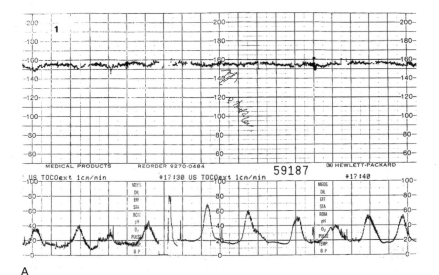

A

Figure 7.5 (A–J) A trace with reduced baseline variability for >90 min is abnormal especially in the presence of shallow decelerations in a non-reactive trace. Sequential traces till the baby's demise are shown

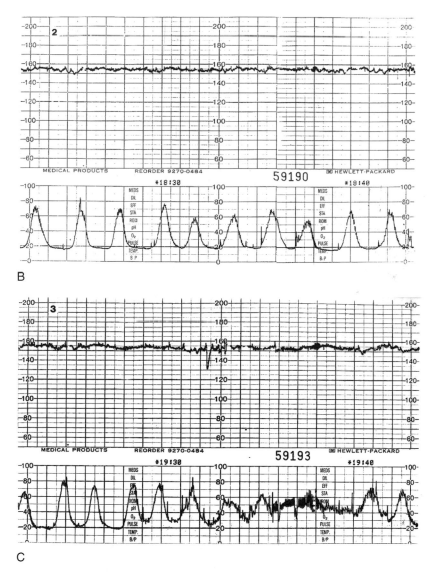

B

C

Figure 7.5 (*continued*)

difficult to know whether the fetus is already hypoxic or acidotic or is suffering from another insult (e.g. infection, brain injury due to haemorrhage, etc.) unless the acid–base status is known prior to or after delivery.

Fetuses with hypoxia may have a normal baseline rate, but with no accelerations, silent pattern (baseline variability below 5) and

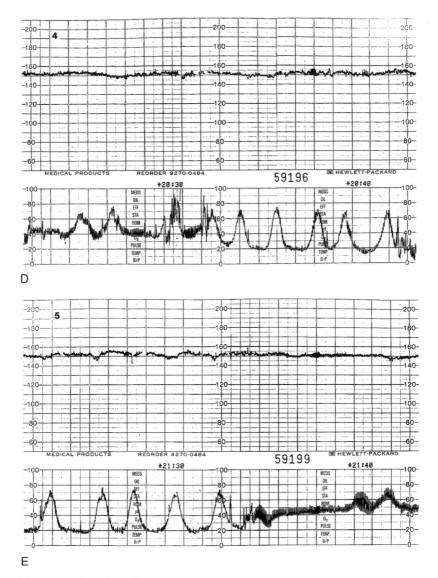

D

E

Figure 7.5 (continued)

shallow decelerations (amplitude less than 15 beats) (see Fig. 7.3). Such a fetus may not stand the stress of labour and may die within 1–2 h of admission. Figure 7.6A–D shows an admission test trace with a baseline rate of 140 bpm. With progress of labour the baseline variability is further reduced (less than 5 beats) without rise in the base-

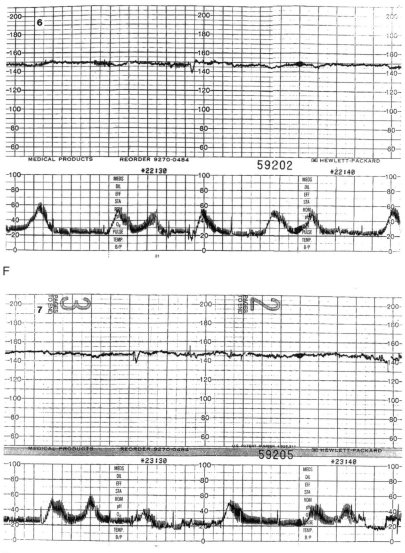

F

G

Figure 7.5 (continued)

line rate and the fetus dies in a span of 40 min. There appears to be some difficulty in identifying the correct baseline rate and some may consider the baseline to be 120 with accelerations. Careful attention to reducing baseline variability would indicate that the correct baseline rate was 140 bpm with decelerations.

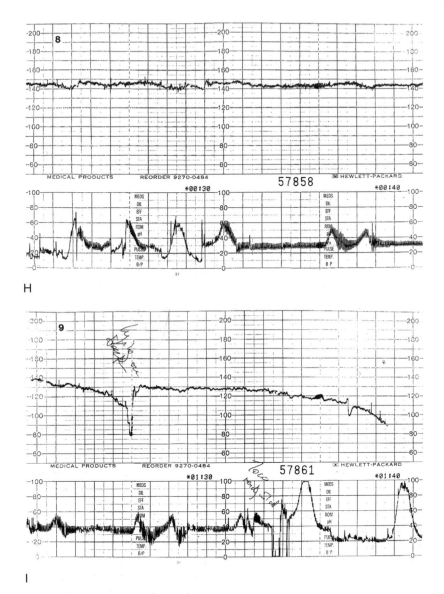

H

I

Figure 7.5 (continued)

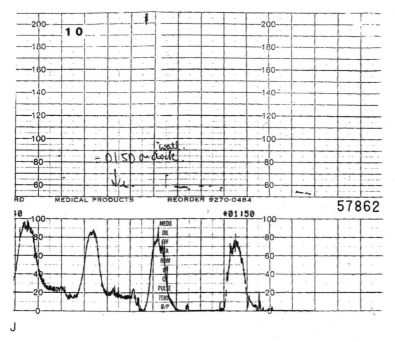

J

Figure 7.5 (continued)

PLANNING MANAGEMENT

An admission test is helpful when planning the subsequent care in labour. High-risk women or women with suspicious or abnormal admission tests should have continuous EFM throughout labour. A normal admission test is an insurance policy that permits us to encourage mobilization with no further need to perform EFM for 3–4 h or until signs of the late first stage of labour are apparent. Even in the second stage of labour a few minutes' strip of EFM after a contraction should be enough in the low-risk woman. Alternative delivery positions, the use of water immersion in labour and preparations for water birth may be more confidently pursued.

A shortage of paper imposes a discipline requiring careful consideration. An admission test followed by monitoring in the late first stage and second stage, the time of greatest stress, appears appropriate.

HOW LONG SHOULD AN ADMISSION TEST LAST?

An AT should last as long as necessary until it is normal. This implies a consideration of fetal sleep and fetal behavioural states. If two

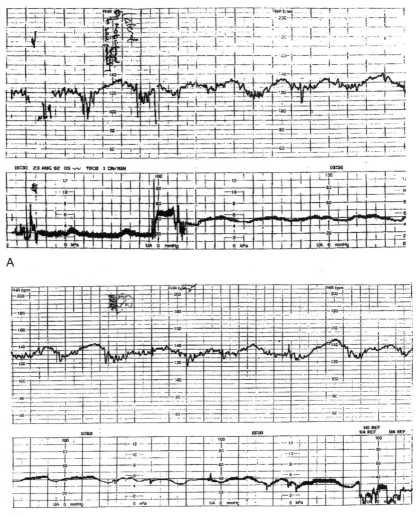

A

B

Figure 7.6 (A–D) A non-reactive trace with normal baseline FHR, silent pattern and shallow decelerations. Sudden fetal demise within 50 min of admission

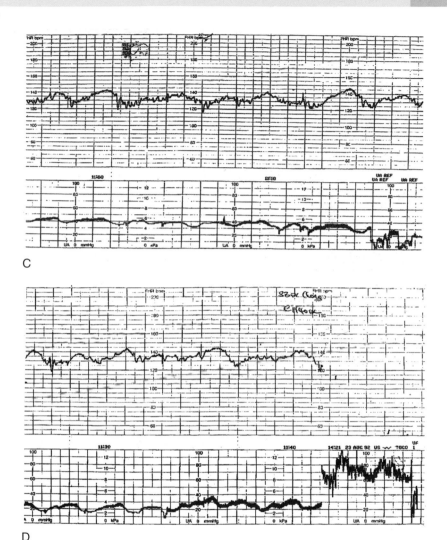

C

D

Figure 7.6 (continued)

accelerations, normal rate and normal variability are seen in the first 5 min then that is very reassuring. It is useful if two or more contractions are witnessed during this time as this will provide reassurance that there is no stress to the fetus with the contractions. If EFM is commenced at the start of a quiescent phase for the fetus then it will need to be continued until the fetus reawakens. Most ATs should last 15–30 min; however, the mother with a normal trace in 5 min, keen for mobilization and natural labour, should not be monitored unduly. Midwives can gain more confidence in the home birth situation by applying these principles and using a hand-held Doptone and, if necessary, a connected printer.

The parents should be given a choice, as in every matter, however the choice provider may find it difficult to offer truly informed choices. It seems to us the simple question that the parents should be asked is 'Would you like us to check that your baby is OK?'

EFM should be appropriate: not too much, not too little.

Chapter 8

Cardiotocographic interpretation: clinical scenarios

MECONIUM-STAINED AMNIOTIC FLUID

The significance of meconium staining of amniotic fluid has often been debated. There are two principal reasons why meconium is passed by the fetus: maturity and fetal compromise.

The incidence of meconium staining of the amniotic fluid increases steadily from 36 weeks to 42 weeks of gestation when it reaches in excess of 20%. This reflects maturation of the central nervous system and gastrointestinal tract manifested by increasing intestinal motility.[77,78] The passage of meconium by a preterm fetus is rare and characteristically associated with the unusual but lethal listerial infection.[55] Fetal compromise, usually of an acute or subacute nature, also leads to the passage of meconium. Very acute stress such as placental abruption or umbilical cord prolapse paradoxically does not often lead to the passage of meconium. There are various degrees of meconium staining, ranging from diluted old meconium which is brownish-yellow to thick, green 'pea soup' meconium. Typically, thick undiluted meconium is seen in a breech presentation for mechanical reasons. Under these circumstances it is interpreted differently from the same appearance in a cephalic presentation. In a cephalic presentation the meconium has to find its way from the fetal anus near the fundus of the uterus to the cervix and vagina: it has to pass through the uterine cavity which is normally filled with a good volume of amniotic fluid; this is the fluid for dilution. If there is little fluid then the meconium cannot become diluted and remains thick. If there is a good volume of fluid a greater degree of wetness occurs after membrane rupture, with thinner meconium. When membrane rupture occurs several days after meconium passage then the meconium is thin and old. If there is no amniotic fluid on rupture of the membranes then concern may be justified on suspicion of oligohydramnios. Thick, fresh meconium in a cephalic presentation suggests oligohydramnios and if the trace is abnormal then delivery should be expedited unless it is expected without delay. In The National Maternity Hospital, Dublin, on every bedside on the labour ward there is a specimen of that woman's amniotic fluid in a universal container. This focuses the attention on the issues involved (Fig. 8.1).

Clear amniotic fluid is reassuring.

Thick, fresh meconium in a situation of high risk is of great concern.

An attempt should be made in all cases with a fetal heart trace not classified as normal to release amniotic fluid from above the presenting part if necessary; this is done by pushing the presenting part gently upwards. If no fluid appears then the possibility of oligohydramnios and potential fetal compromise must be considered.

TWIN PREGNANCY

Perinatal mortality in multiple pregnancy is considerably higher than in singleton pregnancy, and particular risks are present during labour and delivery. It is now known that this mortality is considerably increased for monochorionic twins compared to their dichorionic counterparts. The rare monoamniotic twins should be delivered by caesarean section because of the risk of cord accidents, particularly after the delivery of the first twin. There is an increasing tendency to deliver monochorionic, diamniotic twins by caesarean section because of the risk of acute fetomaternal transfusion. If this

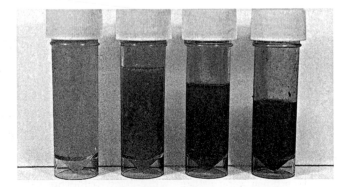

Figure 8.1 Meconium specimens

is not done then very careful electronic monitoring must be undertaken. Twins are generally smaller than singletons, with more pathological growth restriction. The second twin may be at greater risk of this and the ability to electronically monitor both twins continuously is therefore important. The latest generation of fetal monitors have been specially designed to perform this function. One twin can be monitored on direct electrode with the other on ultrasound or both can be monitored using external ultrasound. To have only one machine at a woman's bedside is a considerable advantage which should be fully exploited. The Sonicaid Meridian prints its own paper and therefore has the novel feature of a three channel trace (Fig. 8.2). The Hewlett-Packard and Corometrics models have a technique of printing out both traces in the same channel but in different shades (Fig. 8.3). It is critical to follow the second twin with the ultrasound transducer: this may prove difficult, especially in an obese mother. Assisted delivery is performed for the same indications as in a singleton pregnancy. A senior resident doctor must supervise the delivery of the second twin and ensure continuous electronic fetal monitoring during the interval between deliveries. Such an approach permits a more measured, less anxious delivery process; however, this should not be used as a justification for undue prolongation of the interval.

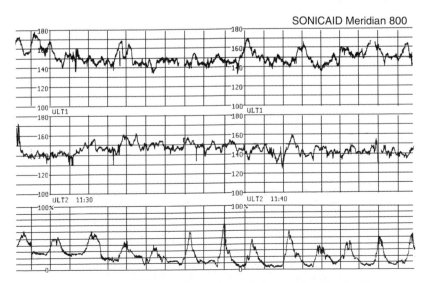

Figure 8.2 Monitoring twins – three channel trace (Oxford Sonicaid Meridian)

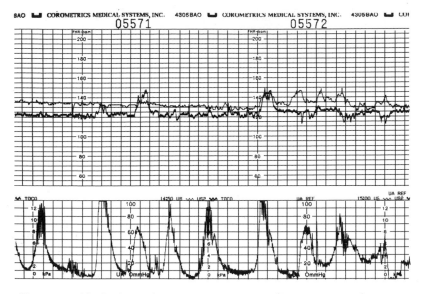

Figure 8.3 Monitoring twins – two channel trace (Corometrics 116)

BREECH PRESENTATION

Babies presenting by the breech are acknowledged to be exposed to more risks than those presenting by the head. The Term Breech Trial Collaborative Group's study has resulted in most breech babies being delivered by caesarean section.[79] This is unfortunate as women who like to deliver vaginally are now being denied the opportunity of vaginal breech birth and doctors in training no longer have the opportunity to acquire this skill.

There are several risks, but intrauterine growth restriction (IUGR) and umbilical cord compression have particular implications for fetal monitoring. The footling or flexed breech has a greater chance of cord prolapse and compression of the umbilical cord in labour. This is a classical scenario for variable decelerations due to cord compression as outlined in Chapter 4. This is one of the reasons why such cases usually have planned caesarean section. There is also evidence that compression of the skull above the orbits by the uterine fundus is a mechanism for variable decelerations. Figure 8.4 shows a typical pattern of cord compression in a breech. Should the misfortune of umbilical cord prolapse occur then the dramatic decelerative pattern shown in Figure 8.5 may be seen. The presence

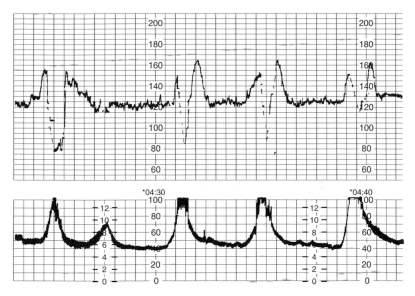

Figure 8.4 Breech presentation: variable decelerations

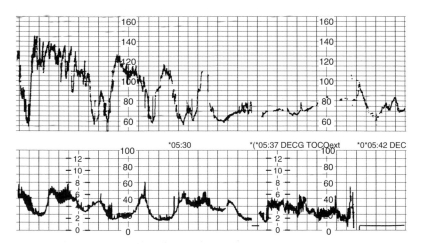

Figure 8.5 Breech cord prolapse

or absence of developing asphyxial features, such as changes in the baseline rate, baseline variability and magnitude of the decelerations related to the speed of the evolving labour process, will relate to the outcome. Breech presentation presents special risks, and in view of these there is little or no place for fetal blood sampling in a breech labour. The blood is more difficult to obtain from the tissues of the breech and it may be different from that obtained from scalp skin. Having understood the normal mechanisms of cardiotocograph (CTG) changes in a breech, if there is a good indication for pH measurement then there is a good indication for caesarean section.

BROW PRESENTATION

Brow presentation in labour in late pregnancy is very unfavourable for vaginal delivery. The mentovertical diameter, which is usually about 13 cm, presents at the pelvic brim. This leads to head compression due to a mechanical misfit. Early and variable decelerations (Fig. 8.6) are associated with this.

There are no typical features associated with a face presentation. The placement of a fetal electrode should be avoided in a recognized face presentation.

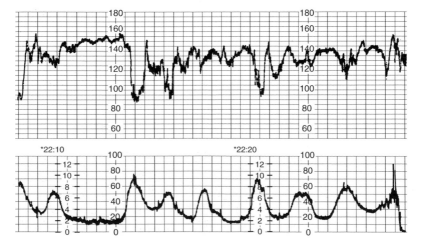

Figure 8.6 Brow presentation: decelerations

PREVIOUS CAESAREAN SECTION: TRIAL OF LABOUR WITH A SCAR

The stability of the placental circulation and uteroplacental perfusion is dependent on the integrity of the uterus and vasculature. With the dehiscence or rupture of the scar, the major uterine blood vessels may become stretched and torn, compromising the perfusion of the placenta (see Fig. 11.4a and b). There is also the possibility of the umbilical cord prolapsing through the dehisced scar, giving rise to a dramatic cord compression pattern (see Fig. 12.1a–f). It is, therefore, believed that changes in the fetal heart rate (FHR) as a result of this may be one of the first signs of scar dehiscence. The other signs of scar dehiscence, such as scar pain, tenderness, vaginal bleeding or alterations in maternal haemodynamics, are notoriously unreliable. Figure 8.7 shows a trace from a woman having a trial of scar where, at laparotomy shortly after the trace, the scar was found to have ruptured. Figure 8.8 shows another trial of labour where emergency caesarean section was undertaken for prolonged bradycardia with a suspicion of scar dehiscence. The baby was delivered by immediate caesarean section (less than 15 min from the decision to delivery), had Apgar scores of 4 at 1 min improving to 7 at 5 min, making a good recovery. There were no signs of placental abruption, scar dehiscence or any other explanation for the bad tracing. Figure 8.9 illustrates another case where the fetus was already passing into the peritoneal cavity with a relatively normal trace and subsequently good outcome. Presumably there was some maintenance of placental perfusion. Continuous electronic FHR monitoring in a trial labour with a scar may be helpful in the diagnosis of scar dehiscence, although this is variable.

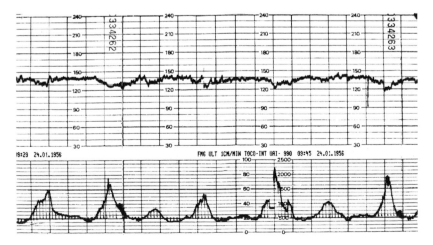

Figure 8.7 Scar rupture: trace with no alarming features

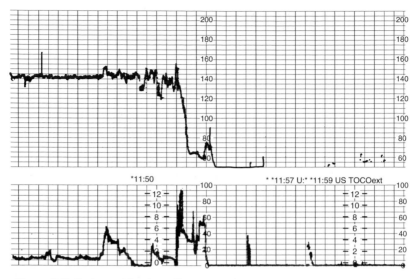

Figure 8.8 Prolonged bradycardia

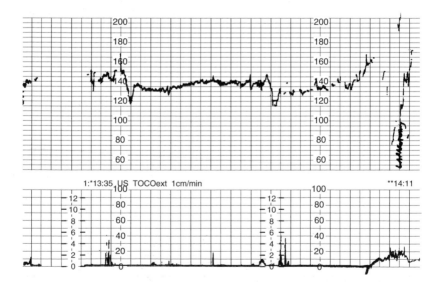

Figure 8.9 Scar rupture: relatively normal trace

SEVERE HYPERTENSION

Women suffering from severe hypertensive disease of pregnancy have at least two possible reasons for having an abnormal CTG. The first is the disease itself and its possible association with IUGR; the second is medication. Antihypertensive drugs, by their very nature, have effects on the maternal and fetal cardiovascular systems. Methyldopa leads to reduction in baseline variability and accelerations. Beta-blocking drugs result in reduced baseline variability and accelerations.[80] Figure 8.10 shows the trace of a fetus whose mother was being treated with labetalol for her hypertension; in spite of numerous fetal movements, accelerations are limited and baseline variability reduced. The picture is confounded by medication in these high-risk pregnancies, and complementary tests such as biophysical profile and Doppler studies are appropriate.

ECLAMPSIA

A convulsion represents a major stress to the fetus which it may not survive. It is likely that such a fetus is already suffering from IUGR because of severe pre-eclampsia. Figure 8.11 shows a trace during an eclamptic fit. After any major acute stress it is important to check fetal condition by ultrasound scan or Doppler transducer of CTG before caesarean section.

The mother's condition must be stabilized before she faces the further challenge of caesarean delivery. If the fetal heart tracing is not

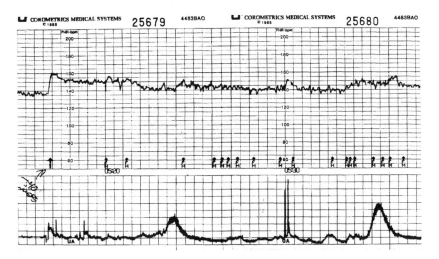

Figure 8.10 Hypertension treated with beta-blocker

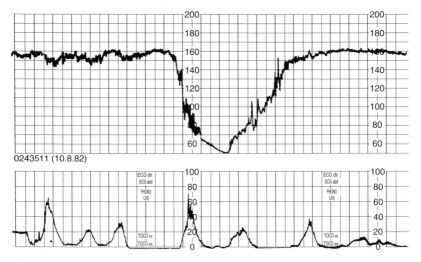

Figure 8.11 Deceleration: eclamptic fit

of major concern after the convulsion then assessment and preparation for 1–2 h is reasonable. Undue haste may lead to maternal complications.

MEDICATION

High-risk women may be on multiple drug therapy. Figure 8.12 shows a trace from a woman with a functioning transplanted kidney who had been prescribed azathioprine, ciclosporin, prednisolone, antibiotics and atenolol. The low baseline is remarkable. Other tests of fetal wellbeing were normal. The trace remained normal in induced labour and the baby was in excellent condition at birth.

A baseline rate below 100 beats per min (bpm) in a non-hypoxic fetus is exceptional.

EPIDURAL ANAESTHESIA

The insertion of an anaesthetic agent into the epidural space can be associated with a degree of instability of the maternal vascular system. Providing the preceding trace has been normal then this represents a stress to the fetus that it can withstand. After attention is paid to the circulating volume, and vascular stability returns, then the trace returns to normal. This is a form of stress test. However, it is wise to apply a scalp electrode before the manipulation for insertion of the epidural to facilitate monitoring, if the preceding trace has not been normal. If the preceding trace has been abnormal then a more ominous

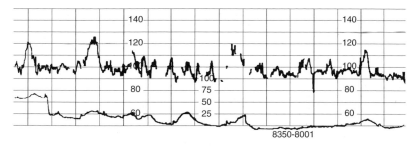

Figure 8.12 Unusual trace: multiple drug therapy

situation may develop. Figure 8.13A is a trace erroneously not recognized to be abnormal before the insertion of the epidural. The cervix was already 3 cm dilated and the trace should have prompted membrane rupture which would have revealed thick meconium and facilitated the application of a scalp electrode. Unfortunately, the stress of epidural insertion resulted in serious asphyxial CTG changes (Fig. 8.13B) and the birth by immediate caesarean section of a compromised baby.

SECOND STAGE OF LABOUR

The second stage is a time of very specific changes in the mechanical effects resulting from descent of the fetus. In a cephalic presentation the initial appearances result from head compression. It is commonly seen in a multiparous mother in good labour that the onset of progressive early decelerations is a sign of the second stage before it has been confirmed by vaginal examination or the appearance of the head at the perineum.

Decelerations are common in the second stage.

Early decelerations gradually becoming deeper and developing variable features are characteristic of the second stage of labour. Reassurance is provided by a good recovery from each deceleration and a return to normal rate and normal variability, however short, before the next contraction (Fig. 8.14). Under these circumstances assisted delivery is not necessary except for other reasons relating to maternal condition. Signs of hypoxia are gradual tachycardia, reduced baseline variability in between and during decelerations (Fig. 8.15), additional late decelerations (Fig. 8.16) and failure of FHR to return to the baseline rate after decelerations (Figs 8.17 and 8.18).[81]

Prolonged bradycardia necessitates delivery.

Failure of the FHR to return to the baseline, and especially failure to recover to at least 100 bpm, is a serious sign and delivery should be undertaken. Figure 8.17 is an example where the doctor was called within 3 min of a bradycardia. At that point the fetal heart then

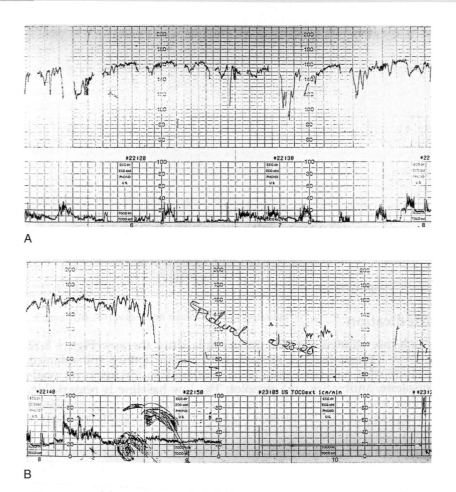

Figure 8.13 (A) Abnormal trace not recognized before insertion of epidural; (B) after epidural, grossly abnormal FHR pattern, leading to operative delivery

recovered. There was a further bradycardia of 3 min which did not then recover. At 6 min the mother was prepared, at 9 min the forceps were prepared and at 12 min the forceps delivery was performed with the baby born in good condition.

The 3, 6, 9 and 12 min rule

- 3 min: call the doctor
- 6 min: prepare the mother

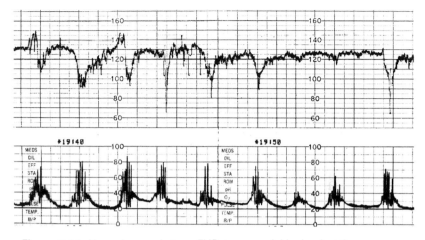

Figure 8.14 Normal second stage FHR trace: variable decelerations

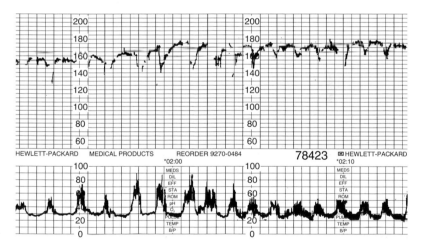

Figure 8.15 Abnormal second stage FHR trace: developing tachycardia

- 9 min: prepare the forceps
- 12 min: deliver the baby.

A delay of 20 min or more may result in an asphyxiated baby.

With a head on or near the perineum one should try to achieve an early delivery. There is no need for washing, gowning, draping and catheterization. A pair of gloves and an instrument such as a Kiwi cup are sufficient. Time is of the essence.

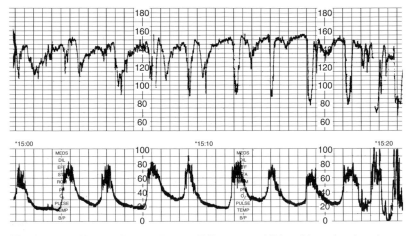

Figure 8.16 Abnormal second stage FHR trace: additional late decelerations

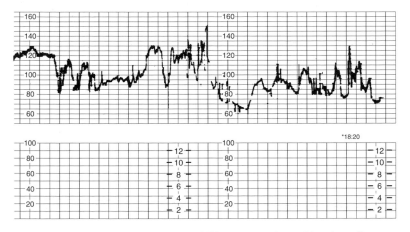

Figure 8.17 Abnormal second stage FHR trace: prolonged bradycardia

PROLONGED DECELERATIONS IN THE FIRST STAGE OF LABOUR

Immediate delivery in this situation will necessitate a caesarean section. There are several publications in the literature that have given the audit findings of the decision to delivery interval, and onset of bradycardia to delivery interval.[82–85] These studies show that in a reasonable proportion of cases delivery was possible by 20 min, and in a further considerable proportion of cases within 30 min. The discussion is related to the possibility of such timings in a busy set up,

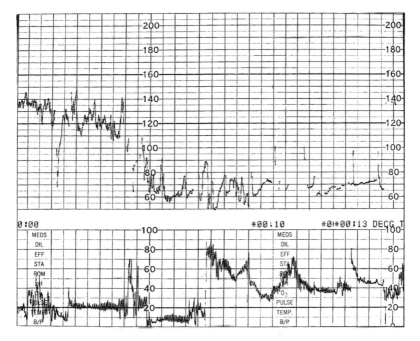

Figure 8.18 Abnormal second stage FHR trace: prolonged bradycardia

especially if the registrar is busy attending to another case. The recommendations of the Royal College of Obstetricians and Gynaecologists to have consultant presence in the labour ward for longer
periods, especially for 24 h in units delivering more than 6000 cases,
may help in such situations.[86] The aim of the teaching of 3, 6, 9, 12
and 15 min guidance (see Ch. 11) is to emphasize the urgency of the
situation in the presence of prolonged decelerations.

Chapter 9

Contraction assessment

Effective contractions (the *powers*) of the uterus are an essential prerequisite for labour and vaginal delivery. The progress of labour, evidenced by dilatation of the uterine cervix and descent of the presenting part, is the final measure of contractions. During the journey through the birth canal (the *passages*), the passenger is intermittently squeezed and stressed by the contractions. Maternal blood flow into the uteroplacental space ceases when the intrauterine pressure (IUP) exceeds the pressure of flow of blood into the retroplacental area, which could be 30–45 mmHg. A well-grown fetus with good placental reserve tolerates this as 'normal stress' and displays no change in the fetal heart rate (FHR). A compromised fetus may show changes with this stress, and reduction of the retroplacental pool of blood due to contractions will be manifested as late decelerations. In a normal fetus, stress can be brought about by cord compression which will be shown as variable decelerations. The presence of atypical variable decelerations indicates that there is cord compression and at the same time there is reduction of retroplacental pool of blood (e.g. atypical variable decelerations with late recovery or a combination of variable and late decelerations). Oxytocin or prostaglandins are given expressly to increase the contractions; when they are given to induce labour the fetus is often already at risk. Particular care should be taken to 'manage' the contractions under these circumstances and to monitor the FHR continuously.

RECORDING

The commonest method of assessing contractions is with the hand placed on the abdominal wall over the anterior part of the uterine fundus. This permits observation of the duration and frequency of contractions. A subjective impression is gained of their strength. This is entirely adequate if performed intermittently in normal low-risk labour.

Continuous monitoring of uterine contractions is performed using external tocography. The tocograph transducer (Fig. 9.1) is a strain gauge device detecting forward movement and change in the abdominal wall contour due to change in shape of the uterus with an anterior thrust on account of the contraction; recording continuously what the hand feels intermittently. The transducer is placed without the application of jelly on the anterior abdominal wall, near the uterine fundus, and secured with an elastic belt. It is important to adjust the tension of the belt for comfort and to secure an adequate recording. Obesity and a restless mother can compromise this. In these circumstances, and in other clinical situations, there may be a role for palpation of uterine contractions or IUP measurement using an intrauterine catheter (Fig. 9.2). IUP measurement is the most effective method of recording contractions including a fairly precise measure of the strength in millimetres of mercury or kilopascals.[87] The technology for this has been developed and several disposable, solid-state devices are available: the Intran II catheter (Fig. 9.3) (Utah Medical Products,

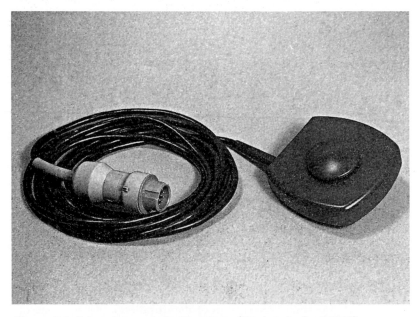

Figure 9.1 External tocography transducer (Hewlett–Packard 8040)

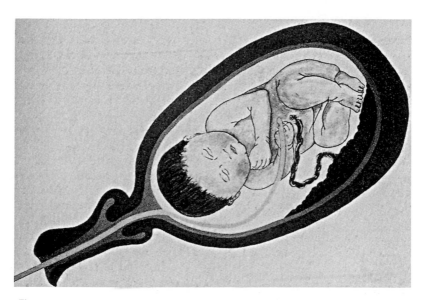

Figure 9.2 Intrauterine catheter in situ

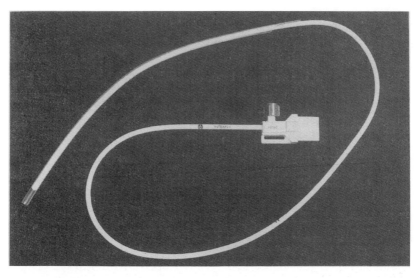

Figure 9.3 Intran II catheter

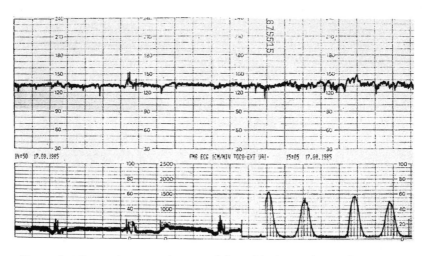

Figure 9.4 External tocography trace followed by internal recording

Utah). Figure 9.4 shows the change in recording in an obese mother seen after converting from external to internal tocography over a period of 20 min.

MEASUREMENT

What are normal contractions? The most relevant measure of contractions in labour is their outcome: dilatation of the cervix and descent of the presenting part resulting in spontaneous vaginal delivery. The quality of contractions present is very variable. A simple assessment of the frequency of contractions (number per 10 min), the mean duration (in seconds) and a subjective impression of strength (weak, moderate or strong) usually suffices. The method of recording this is seen on the partogram (see Fig. 2.3). When IUP monitoring is being used the opportunity arises for greater precision. In 1957 Caldeyro-Barcia suggested Montevideo units using average pressure multiplied by frequency.[88] In 1973 Hon and Paul introduced the concept of contraction area under the curve: uterine activity units.[89] In 1977 Steer introduced the active contractions area under the curve: kilopascal seconds per 15 min.[90] A simple system based on Systeme Internationale (SI) units has been considered and recommended by the Royal College of Obstetrics and Gynaecologists Working Party on Cardiotocograph Technology.[91]

The appropriate units for IUP quantification are listed in Table 9.1, and the appropriate units for measuring the total activity over a

Table 9.1 Units for intrauterine pressure quantification

Mean contraction active pressure (MCAP)	kPa
Mean baseline pressure	kPa
Mean contraction frequency	number per 10 min
Mean duration of contractions	seconds
Mean active pressure (MAP): sum of MCAP divided by time	kPa

Table 9.2 Units for measuring the total activity over a period of time

Active pressure integral (API)	kPa
Baseline pressure integral (BPI)	kPa
Number of contractions per period	
Total duration of contractions	seconds
Proportion of active time	per cent

period of time are listed in Table 9.2. The recommended period of measurement is 15 min.

Consistent terminology is essential.

CLINICAL APPLICATION

What are the indications for continuous tocography? In general, continuous external tocography is performed when continuous FHR monitoring is being performed. This is a pragmatic, practical approach, however it ignores the rationale that the indication for each is separate although they may be related. If the FHR pattern is normal and the labour progress is normal then continuous tocography does not provide additional useful information, and the woman could be spared the discomfort of the tocography belt. There remains the issue that if the fetal heart pattern or labour progress becomes abnormal then information is already available about the pre-existing contractions which are of importance. Hence the 2-channel monitoring – the heart rate and the contractions – is standard. Whenever the heart rate is abnormal or labour progress is abnormal requiring treatment, the need for continuous contraction recording is clear.

Figure 9.5 shows an admission test performed on a woman with tightenings. Although the tocographic tracing suggests frequent

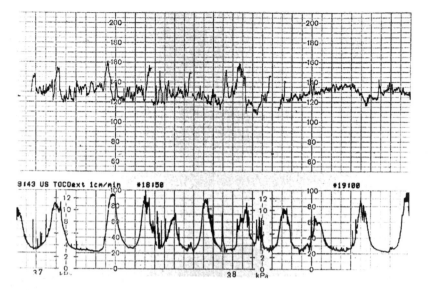

Figure 9.5 Contractions recorded: subject not in labour

regular contractions, the woman was not experiencing pain and did not go into labour that day. The tocography transducer may detect localized contractions that are not propagating throughout the uterus as also shown with marked irregularity in Figure 9.6.

The diagnosis of labour is not made from the cardiotocograph.

What are the indications for internal tocography using an IUP catheter? Other than in an obese or restless mother, external tocography provides enough information to interpret an abnormal fetal heart tracing. The management of the contractions is another issue. If induction of labour or augmentation of slow labour (see Fig. 2.3) is non-progressive then the more complete information derived from an IUP catheter might be useful.[92] However, available data suggest that, in most of these situations, titration of the oxytocin infusion rate based on frequency and duration of contractions recorded by external tocography is adequate.[93,94] The exception might be the obese, restless mother or the nullipara with an occipitoposterior position with poor progress of labour requiring a high-dose infusion of oxytocin.

Breech presentation in labour, nowadays very uncommon, and labour with a previous caesarean section scar present specific problems. Some obstetricians do not practice vaginal delivery of a baby presenting by the breech; in those that do there is some reluctance to use oxytocin if labour progress is slow. The anxiety is that the slow progress is a manifestation of fetopelvic disproportion and therefore the sign to terminate the labour by performing a caesarean section.

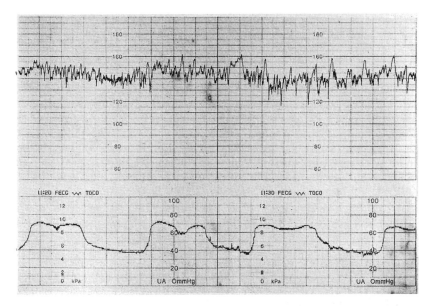

Figure 9.6 Contractions recorded: subject not in labour

The counter-view is that poor contractions are just as likely (if not more likely) to occur in a breech presentation. If complete assessment of the fetopelvic relationship has shown favourable features and the contractions are shown to be weak then oxytocin augmentation may be safely undertaken. The additional information derived from an IUP catheter may be useful under these circumstances.

A similar rationale applies to poor labour progress in a woman with a previous caesarean section scar. Additionally there is the further concern for the integrity of the uterine scar. Scar rupture or dehiscence may not manifest scar pain, tenderness, vaginal bleeding or alteration in maternal pulse and blood pressure or may manifest some time after the event; FHR or uterine activity changes may be an earlier sign of scar disruption.[95,96] Figure 9.7 shows a case where re-siting of the catheter led to an acceptable tocographic tracing in spite of scar dehiscence; presumably the replaced catheter was in a loculated pocket of normal pressure. In some centres there is a link between the indication for internal FHR monitoring with an electrode and internal pressure monitoring with a pressure catheter. There is no logic in this as each addresses separate issues. Excessive use of internal monitoring is invasive psychologically as well as physically.

There is a very limited place for IUP measurement.

Uterine hyperstimulation and fetal hypoxia are a real possibility when oxytocics are used and, in these circumstances, continuous

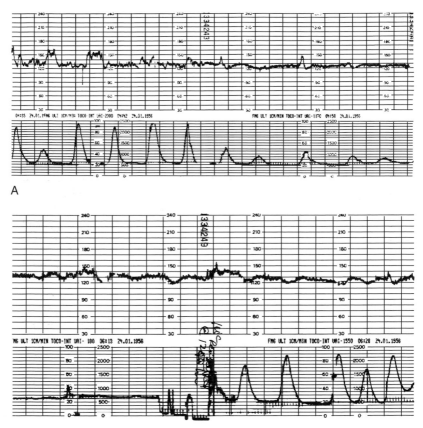

A

B

Figure 9.7 (A) Scar dehiscence: reduction in uterine activity; (B) intrauterine pressure catheter replaced in another pocket showing normal uterine activity

electronic FHR monitoring is important and this is discussed in Chapter 10.

CONTRACTION MONITORING WITH THE USE OF PROSTAGLANDINS FOR INDUCTION OF LABOUR

It is important to record uterine contractions and the FHR prior to, and soon after, insertion of vaginal prostaglandin (PG) pessaries or gels. The rate of absorption of PG varies from woman to woman based on the pH, temperature and moisture content of the vagina and whether there is infection, inflammation or abrasion in the vagina.

Rapid absorption can give rise to tetanic or too frequent contractions which need not be painful but may cause suspicious/abnormal FHR changes, including prolonged deceleration that may compromise the fetus if prompt action is not taken. Action can be in the form of removing the PG pessary if possible and/or use of tocolytic agents to abolish uterine contractions.

CONTRACTION MONITORING AFTER EXTERNAL CEPHALIC VERSION

A small abruption leading to uterine irritability and FHR changes may occur following external cephalic version (ECV) without much pain, and hence the need to monitor uterine contractions and the FHR for 30–60 min after ECV. If uterine irritability is observed with too frequent contractions (>5 in 10 min), the FHR may become abnormal and hence the recording should be continued until no, or infrequent, uterine contractions are observed and the FHR pattern is normal.

CONTRACTION MONITORING IN CASES OF SUSPECTED ABRUPTION

In the presence of features suggestive of abruption, i.e. bleeding and/or continuous abdominal pain if there is uterine irritability, uterine contractions and the FHR should be monitored. Consideration should be given for early delivery if the FHR trace is unsatisfactory with uterine irritability, if fetal maturity is not a major concern. In the presence of uterine irritability and suspicious or pathological FHR pattern, the FHR can suddenly deteriorate leading to the need for an emergency delivery.

The development of clinical skills and an educational motive remain important reasons for giving due attention to the contractions. In the USA many cases of litigation relate to the misuse of oxytocin. Better understanding of the labour process and contractions should help to counter such misuse.[97]

Chapter 10

Oxytocin and fetal heart rate changes

Oxytocin is commonly used for induction and augmentation of labour. Many medico-legal cases relate to the misuse of oxytocin. Oxytocin does not have a direct influence on the fetal heart rate (FHR) or on the controlling cardiac centres in the brain, as is the case with some anaesthetic and antihypertensive drugs. Its influence is indirect via increased uterine activity, mostly due to increased frequency of contractions or baseline pressure (hypertonus). Increase in duration or amplitude of contractions can also lead to FHR changes. The NICE guidelines define hyperstimulation as more than five contractions in 10 min (some literature defines it as polysystole) and if it is associated with FHR changes it is defined as 'hyperstimulation syndrome'.[98] Figure 10.1 shows fetal bradycardia due to 'tetanic' or sustained contractions lasting for 3–4 min, caused by oxytocin hyperstimulation. Because the subject was a healthy fetus with a normal reactive FHR prior to the episode, the transient bradycardia returned to normal once the oxytocin infusion was reduced and the abnormal contractions ceased.

Figure 10.2 shows fetal bradycardia due to 'hypertonic' uterine activity. The baseline pressure was elevated by 15 mmHg for 3 min despite regular contractions. The raised baseline pressure reduced the perfusion in the retroplacental area leading to FHR changes, which returned to normal once the baseline pressure settled to normal levels, restoring normal perfusion.

Figure 10.3 shows a reactive trace with one contraction in 3 min. An oxytocin infusion was commenced 10 min from the start of this segment at a rate of 1 mU per min. This resulted in the late decelerations and changes seen in the latter part of the trace. The contraction recording shows no increase in frequency or duration of contractions nor increase in baseline pressure, but shows an increase in amplitude of contractions. Discontinuation of the infusion resulted in return of the FHR trace to normal.

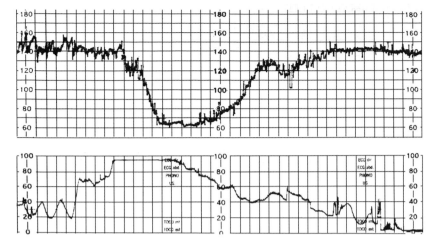
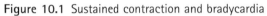

Figure 10.1 Sustained contraction and bradycardia

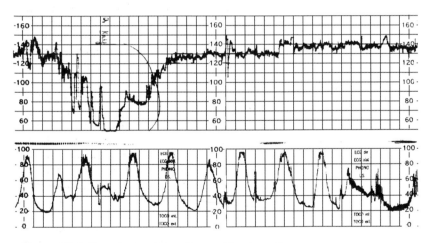
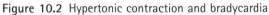

Figure 10.2 Hypertonic contraction and bradycardia

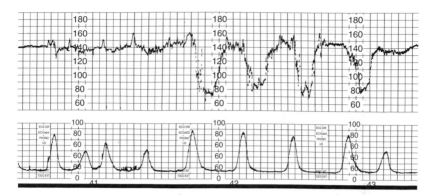

Figure 10.3 Normal trace and subsequent decelerations with oxytocin

The FHR changes associated with oxytocin infusion may be caused by compression of the cord with contractions or by the reduction in placental perfusion due to increased intrauterine basal pressure and frequent contractions cutting off the blood supply to the placenta. Pressure on the head or supraorbital region of the fetus can also give rise to variable decelerations. The rate of increasing hypoxia would be shown by a deteriorating trend of the FHR. The rate of decline of pH depends on the FHR pattern observed and the physiological reserve of the fetus.[99] A rapid decline would be anticipated in post-term and growth-restricted fetuses and those with reduced amniotic fluid with thick meconium, infection or intrapartum bleeding. Fortunately, in the vast majority of patients who are given oxytocin, FHR changes of a worrying nature are not encountered and most changes, even when they occur, are transient and resolve spontaneously, or with reduction of the dose or transient cessation of the infusion. It is good practice to run a strip of cardiotocograph prior to commencing oxytocin to make sure of good fetal health as reflected by a normal reactive FHR pattern: *if the trace is pathological then oxytocin should not be used*, as it can cause further hypoxia to the fetus by reducing the perfusion to the placenta by additional contractions.

If a pathological FHR pattern is observed in a woman on an oxytocin infusion, the infusion should be stopped, or its rate reduced, and the woman nursed on her side to improve the maternal venous return, and thus her cardiac output, in order to increase the utero-placental perfusion. Oxygen inhalation by the mother and an intravenous bolus of tocolytic drugs to abolish uterine contractions are given in some centres. Such practice may not be necessary in the majority of cases and its value in other cases is debatable. It is known that oxytocin becomes bound to receptors, and for its action to be reduced to half can take up to 45 min after stopping the oxytocin infusion. A case may be made for the use of a bolus dose of a tocolytic drug in a patient with a grossly abnormal (pathological) FHR pattern.[100,101] There is little merit in performing a fetal scalp blood pH measurement in a patient receiving oxytocin since the FHR changes are iatrogenic. If the test is done soon after a prolonged bradycardia, or after ominous decelerations, it may show acidosis prompting the performance of an emergency caesarean section (Fig. 10.4A). On

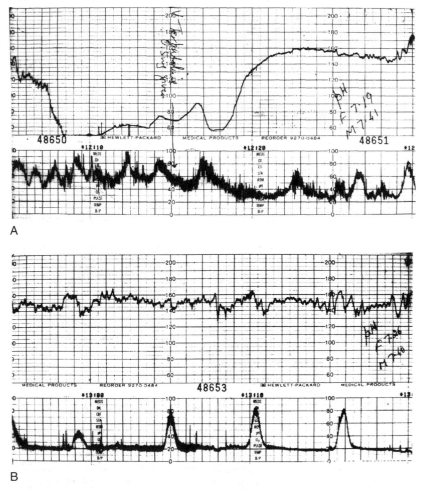

A

B

Figure 10.4 (A) Cardiotocograph: bradycardia with acidosis and (B) reversion to normal pH the other hand, if a fetal blood sample is not taken and time is allowed, the FHR recovers and within 30–40 min the scalp blood pH is likely to be normal (Fig. 10.4B). On many occasions there is no need to measure scalp blood pH and the oxytocin infusion can be restarted after the return of the FHR to normal.

It is debatable for how long the oxytocin infusion should be stopped once the FHR abnormality is detected. It is usual to wait until the abnormal features disappear and the reactive trace is seen; however, it is known that although the trace is then normal, the fetal blood biochemistry reflected on scalp blood testing may still show a low pH, high PCO_2 and low PO_2. Additional time is required for the blood biochemistry to become normal, which takes place rapidly once the FHR is normal. Noting the time necessary for the FHR to become normal after the oxytocin infusion is stopped, and allowing an equal length of time to elapse before restarting the infusion, would allow the biochemistry to become normal. Doubling the time period in this way before restarting oxytocin should cause little or no FHR changes compared with restarting oxytocin immediately after the FHR returns to normal. It is also advisable to resume the infusion at half the previous dose rate to reduce the chances of hyperstimulation or abnormal FHR changes. Since the sensitivity of the uterus to oxytocin increases with progress of labour,[102] such careful titration is likely to produce fewer problems of abnormal FHR changes or uterine hyperstimulation. Increased uterine activity in the late first stage and second stage of labour may be due to reflex release of oxytocin due to distension of the cervix and the upper vagina, i.e. the Ferguson reflex.[103]

Figure 10.5A shows abnormal FHR changes produced by oxytocic hyperstimulation. Even with immediate cessation of oxytocin infusion it takes about 45 min for the FHR to return to normal (Fig. 10.5B) and hence sufficient time should be given for recovery. Although it is advisable to stop the oxytocin infusion as soon as abnormal FHR patterns, such as decelerations or bradycardia, are observed, it may be adequate to reduce the oxytocin dose by half or less when the FHR is normal but there is abnormal uterine activity.

Figure 10.6A shows a reactive FHR at the beginning, but decelerations and tachycardia subsequently develop owing to increased frequency of contractions. In Figure 10.6B the FHR becomes tachycardic: towards the latter part of the trace, the dose of oxytocin was reduced to half and the tocographic transducer was adjusted. In Figure 10.6c the contractions have become less frequent, the FHR has settled to a normal baseline rate and is followed by a reactive pattern.

In cases of failure to progress in labour, oxytocin is commenced to augment uterine contractions. This may bring about FHR changes when the dose is increased to achieve the optimal target frequency of contractions. If the dose is reduced, the FHR pattern returns to normal

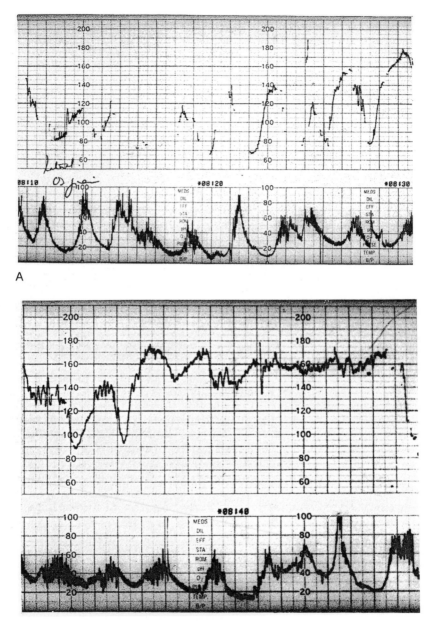

A

B

Figure 10.5 (A) Hyperstimulation and abnormal trace followed by (B) correction of trace after cessation of oxytocin

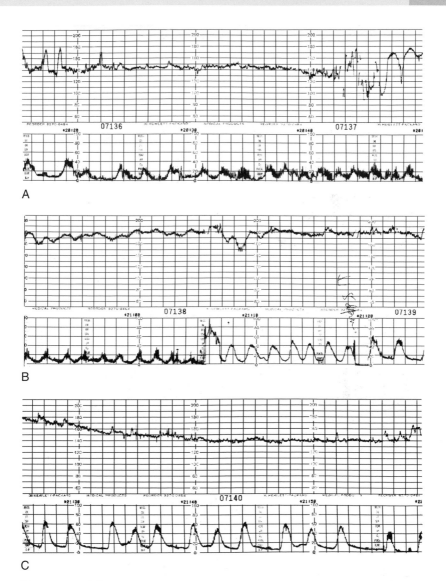

Figure 10.6 (A) Increased frequency of contractions: changes in trace; (B) sustained tachycardia; (C) reversion to normal after reduction of oxytocin

but the uterine activity drops to suboptimal levels with no progress in labour. When FHR changes are encountered in such a situation, they may be transient and it may be worth stopping and restarting oxytocin or reducing the dose. However, if pathological FHR changes appear when oxytocin is recommenced despite these efforts, it may be better to deliver abdominally. In selected cases further time may be given to see whether the labour will progress without the use of oxytocin. An alternative would be to stop oxytocin and perform a fetal blood sample 20–30 min later and, if the pH is normal, to restart the oxytocin infusion and observe for any rise in the baseline rate and/or reduction of baseline variability. In the absence of these changes or in the absence of increase of the width or depth of the decelerations a cervical assessment can be made to assess progress in 1–2 h time. If there is no progress caesarean section may be appropriate. If there is adequate progress a repeat pH can be performed. The rate of decline of pH related to the rate of progress of cervical dilatation can be deduced and a decision made to allow progress if the pH is unlikely to be acidotic by the time of anticipated delivery. Obviously the plans need to be changed if there is a worsening FHR pattern.

In induced labour, in the absence of disproportion, the uterus has to perform a certain amount of uterine activity depending on the parity and cervical score to achieve vaginal delivery. Considering this, it may be possible to achieve optimal uterine activity which does not cause FHR changes but is adequate to bring about slow but progressive cervical dilatation.[92] The labour may be a little longer, during which time adequate contractions are generated to achieve vaginal delivery. However, such management needs intrauterine catheters and equipment to compute uterine activity, and it may not be possible to achieve optimal uterine activity without FHR changes and achieve vaginal delivery.

MEDICO-LEGAL CONSIDERATIONS

The major concerns with oxytocin and medico-legal issues relate to the following:

- Inadequate uterine contraction monitoring.
- Poor technical quality of the FHR trace.
- Cessation of monitoring the FHR or uterine contractions much earlier than the time of delivery.
- Commencement of oxytocin when there are major risk factors, e.g. thick meconium-stained scanty fluid, evidence of chorioamnionitis and a suspicious or abnormal FHR trace.
- Failure to recognize that the uterus is contracting >5 in 10 min despite no increase in oxytocin infusion and failure to reduce or

stop the oxytocin infusion, thereby causing a pathological FHR pattern such as prolonged decelerations and fetal compromise.

- Failure to use tocolytics in some cases to alleviate the problem early, as time is needed for oxytocin-induced contractions to reduce/abate.
- Failure to recognize that prolonged decelerations may follow a normal FHR trace and it may not recover despite stopping oxytocin if the FHR prior to the decelerations was suspicious or abnormal.
- When prolonged decelerations occur the fetal monitor may record the 'maternal heart rate' which may not be recognized by the caregiver.
- The fetus may be affected with hypoxia despite prompt action (e.g. delivery) but the caregiver may be liable if the prolonged FHR decelerations were caused by uterine hyperstimulation.
- Oxytocin should be used with caution when there are FHR changes as it may make things worse. Careful consideration should be given to deliver rather than to augment or induce labour.
- In the presence of thick meconium and scanty fluid, meconium aspiration syndrome is a possibility with late or atypical decelerations suggestive of hypoxia even without acidosis.
- Decelerations in early labour, or prolonged decelerations with the use of oxytocin may imply impending scar rupture with oxytocin in a woman with a previous scar.
- If the FHR shows what appears like accelerations, they may be decelerations if the baseline rate does not settle and show 'active and quiet sleep cyclicity' pattern with continuation of the recording for two hours.

Chapter 11

Cardiotocographic interpretation: more difficult problems

Specific situations that are of specific concern and interest include prolonged deceleration (bradycardia), placental abruption, sinusoidal pattern, the infected fetus, the abnormal fetus and the dying fetus. In recent times, inadvertent recording of the maternal heart rate (MHR) mimicking the fetal heart rate (FHR) that has not been recognized by staff has led to adverse outcomes, and this is also discussed here.

PROLONGED DECELERATION (BRADYCARDIA)

Prolonged FHR deceleration (bradycardia) (FHR <80 beats per min (bpm)) for less than 3 min is considered suspicious, and for greater than 3 min is regarded as abnormal. A deceleration of greater than 3 min could be due to an acute event and may be a warning signal of acute hypoxia due to cord compression or prolapse, abruptio placentae, scar dehiscence, uterine hyperstimulation or another unknown cause. It can occur in healthy fetuses (possibly due to cord compression). Reversible causes for such an episode are epidural top up, vaginal examination and uterine hyperstimulation. Simple measures such as adjusting maternal position, stopping the oxytocin infusion, attending to hydration and giving oxygen by face mask may correct the condition. A patient who presents with continuous abdominal pain, vaginal bleeding, a tender, tense or irritable uterus and prolonged fetal bradycardia is likely to have suffered an abruption and warrants immediate delivery. Those in whom scar dehiscence or rupture is suspected, and those with cord prolapse, may present with prolonged bradycardia and need immediate delivery.

Most cases of prolonged bradycardia with no major pathology will show signs of recovery towards the baseline rate within 6 min.

If the clinical picture does not suggest abruption, scar dehiscence or cord prolapse, and if the fetus is appropriately grown at term with clear amniotic fluid and a reactive FHR pattern prior to the episode of bradycardia, return back to the baseline FHR pattern within 9 min is to be expected. The recovery towards the normal baseline within 6 min with good baseline variability at the time of the bradycardia and during recovery are reassuring signs, and one should wait with confidence that the FHR will revert to the normal baseline with a normal pattern. If there are no signs of recovery towards the baseline rate by 6 min, action should be taken to determine the cause, to determine cervical dilatation and to consider delivery. If the cervix is fully dilated and the head is low, a forceps or ventouse delivery should be carried out, but a caesarean section may be preferred if the cervix is not fully dilated or the head is high. This caesarean section comes under category 1 or grade 1 in terms of the classification for the urgency with which it should be done. Category 1 should have a specific code or term assigned, such as 'grade 1', 'code red' or 'immediate', 'emergency' or 'crash' caesarean section, in order to mobilize all the staff (obstetricians, anaesthetists, additional midwifery staff, theatre staff, operating department assistants and paediatricians) needed to accomplish delivering the baby within 30 min of the decision being made. Obviously the decision should be made as early as possible but without overreaction. The best policy may be for the midwife and the doctor in that room to push the bed to the theatre while the midwife on duty calls for the anaesthetist, paediatric and theatre staff. Early entry into the theatre offers the opportunity for more people to help with the various tasks of setting up an IV line, sending blood for Hb and 'group and save', catheterization, and explaining to the couple the need for caesarean section and reassuring them.

A 45-year-old multiparous woman was well known to the medical staff and midwives. A diagnosis of term labour was made at 22.00 h when the cervix was 5 cm dilated and the initial cardiotocograph (CTG) was normal (Fig. 11.1A). Shortly before midnight a prolonged bradycardia became manifest after an otherwise normal trace (Fig. 11.1B). The midwife correctly annotated 'FH' at the end of this strip of trace. Figure 11.1C shows the heart rate improving with good variability; however, the inexperienced obstetric registrar decided to perform a caesarean section and consequently the trace shows 'discontinued for theatre'. Not surprisingly the Apgar scores were 9 at 1 min and 10 at 5 min. If the trace had not been disconnected it would have reverted to normal; a premature decision led to an unnecessary caesarean section in a multiparous woman in whom labour was probably progressing rapidly. A longer contraction duration or transient cord compression might

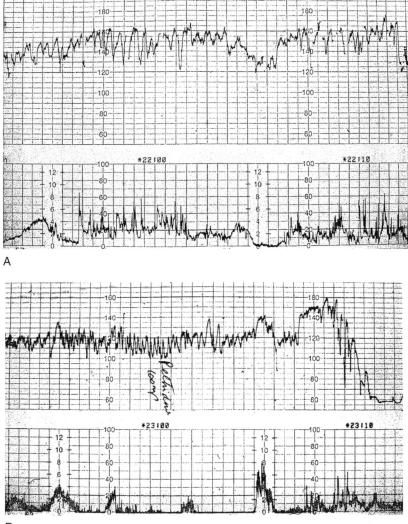

Figure 11.1 (A) Cardiotocograph: normal reactive pattern; (B) Prolonged bradycardia

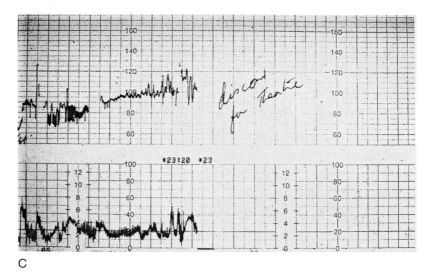

C

Figure 11.1 (*continued*) (C) Improvement in heart rate

account for the deceleration. The diagnosis was 'obstetric registrar's distress'!

If the FHR does not show signs of recovery by 9 min the incidence of acidosis is increased, and one should take action to deliver the fetus as soon as possible.[100] The clinical picture has to be considered while anxiously awaiting the FHR to return to normal. Fetuses who are post term, growth restricted, have no amniotic fluid or have thick meconium-stained fluid at rupture of membranes are at a greater risk of developing hypoxia. Those with an abnormal or suspicious FHR trace prior to the episode of bradycardia are also at a greater risk of hypoxia developing within a short time. In these situations it may be better to take action early if the FHR fails to return to normal. If uterine hyperstimulation due to oxytocics is the cause, oxytocin infusion should be stopped. Inhibition of uterine contractions with a bolus intravenous dose of a betamimetic drug may be of value in some situations. Fetal scalp blood sampling (FBS) at the time of persistent prolonged deceleration, or soon after, may delay urgently needed action and is contraindicated.[13] Figure 11.2 shows the trace in a case without obvious risk factors. Fetal scalp blood sampling, which can prolong the deceleration due to pressure on the fetal head, delayed delivery. Caesarean section was eventually performed. The baby had very poor Apgar scores and died on the third day after a period of neonatal convulsions.

Fetal acidosis observed soon after a prolonged deceleration (Fig. 11.3A) will recover when the trace returns to normal (Fig. 11.3B).

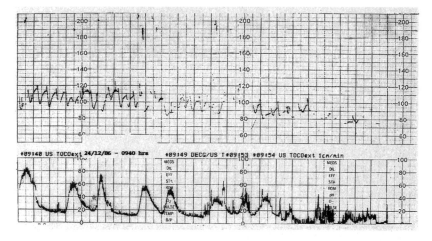

Figure 11.2 Fetal scalp blood sampling delays delivery: poor outcome

Alternatively, if the fetal heart rate does not return to normal, delivery should be undertaken. During a prolonged deceleration the fetus reduces its cardiac output. Carbon dioxide and other metabolites cannot be cleared by the respiratory function of the placenta. The initial pH at the end of a prolonged deceleration is low with a high PCO_2 showing a respiratory acidosis. Once the FHR returns to normal the carbon dioxide and metabolites are cleared and the pH and blood gases return to normal in 30–40 min. If the episode of prolonged deceleration continues then the fetus switches to anaerobic metabolism resulting in metabolic acidosis which is harmful to the fetus. Hence excessively prolonged deceleration results in a poor outcome.

Scalp pH measurement should not be performed for prolonged deceleration.

Scar rupture or dehiscence may not show the classical symptoms and signs of scar pain, tenderness, vaginal bleeding or alteration in maternal pulse or blood pressure. Changes in FHR or uterine activity may be an earlier manifestation of loss of integrity of the scar, and prompt action should avoid fetal or maternal morbidity or mortality. In these cases a prolonged deceleration may be an ominous sign and may indicate scar rupture. Figure 11.4A shows a prolonged deceleration in a case of labour with a previous caesarean section. Delivery was delayed (Fig. 11.4B), resulting in a baby with poor Apgar scores and neonatal asphyxial death on the second day. Whenever an operative delivery is planned the fetal heart should be checked prior to delivery as the baby may be already dead if there has been delay. In one such case prolonged deceleration followed an eclamptic fit

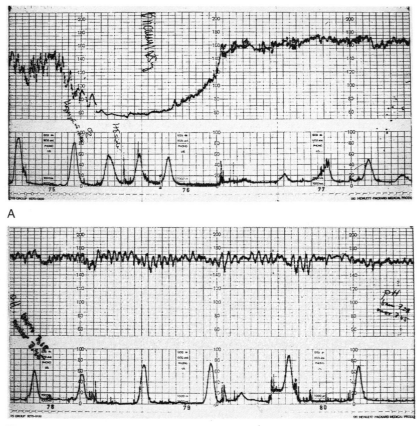

A

B

Figure 11.3 (A) Acidosis at time of bradycardia; (B) pH recovers after trace returns to normal

(Fig. 11.5). The convulsions were controlled and the baby was delivered in 30 min; a reasonable delay to stabilize the maternal condition. The fetal heart was not verified just before delivery and the baby was a fresh stillbirth.[104] In cases of placental abruption it may not be possible to listen to the fetal heart with a stethoscope or an electronic monitor. An ultrasound scan is therefore useful.

The procedure in the case of prolonged deceleration is shown in Table 11.1. Each hospital should have facilities to perform an immediate caesarean section and deliver the baby within 15–20 min of taking the decision, especially if high-risk labours (such as cases of previous caesarean section) are being looked after. This is referred to as delivery from a 'hot start'. Delivery by caesarean section from a 'cold start' may be permitted with a decision-to-delivery interval of 30 min. Audit and review of this in any unit is important.

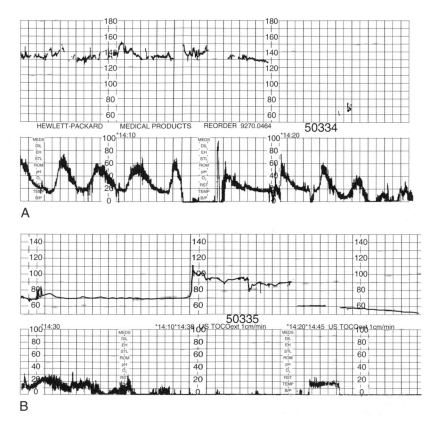

Figure 11.4 (A) Labour with previous caesarean section: prolonged bradycardia; (B) delay in delivery leading to poor outcome

PLACENTAL ABRUPTION

Figure 11.6 shows the initial trace in a woman having induction for proteinuric pregnancy-induced hypertension at term. The fundosymphysis height was 36 cm at 40 weeks' gestation. Initially there is a slightly fast baseline rate with good variability but no accelerations (Fig. 11.6A). A prostaglandin pessary was given and the initial contraction tracing is unremarkable. Forty minutes later the patient complained of increasing pain and restlessness. The tocographic tracing (Fig. 11.6B) shows very frequent contractions of low amplitude which are typical of the irritable uterus in placental abruption. The FHR proceeded to a tachycardia with no further accelerations and with reduced baseline variability and a deceleration (Fig. 11.6C). The woman suffered increasing pain, restlessness and maternal tachycardia. There was no revealed bleeding; however, a clinical impression of placental abruption was clear. As the woman was

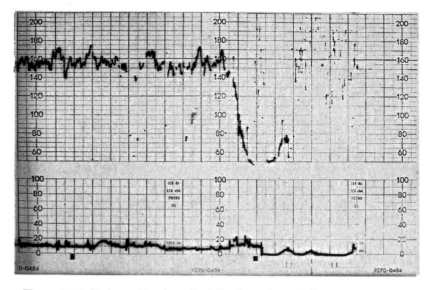

Figure 11.5 Prolonged bradycardia following eclamptic fit

Table 11.1 Procedure for prolonged bradycardia

3 min	Draw attention and review clinical picture and prior FHR trace
6 min	Expect recovery of FHR towards the baseline
9 min	If no recovery, prepare for operative delivery
12 min	Operative procedure should have started
15 min	Baby is delivered

---

being prepared for caesarean section, the FHR dropped abruptly to a bradycardia (Fig. 11.6D). Immediate caesarean section resulted in a moderately asphyxiated baby weighing 2.6 kg who made a good recovery. There was a large retroplacental blood clot.

Frequent low-amplitude contractions and an abnormal CTG trace suggest placental abruption.

SINUSOIDAL FETAL HEART RATE PATTERN

Sinusoidal FHR pattern is a description given to a trace with a sinusoidal waveform appearance. Because of its association with severe anaemia or hypoxic fetuses it is looked upon with anxiety. It is important to realize that severely anaemic fetuses do not always show sinusoidal pattern and that sinusoidal pattern can be exhibited by healthy fetuses at certain times. A typical 'pathological' sinusoidal FHR pattern should

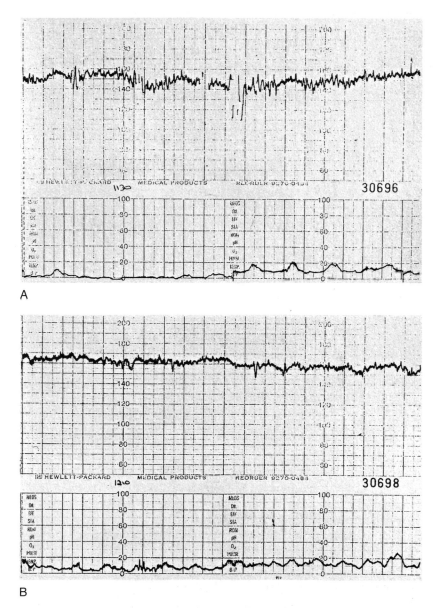

A

B

Figure 11.6 Induction for hypertension: (A) initial trace; (B) frequent low-amplitude contractions, abnormal trace

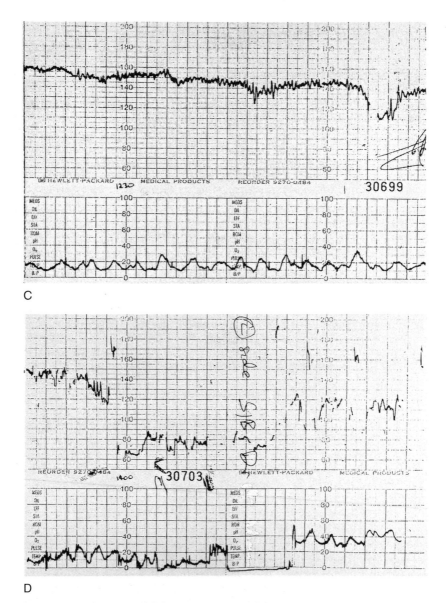

C

D

Figure 11.6 (*continued*) (C) Abnormal trace; (D) bradycardia

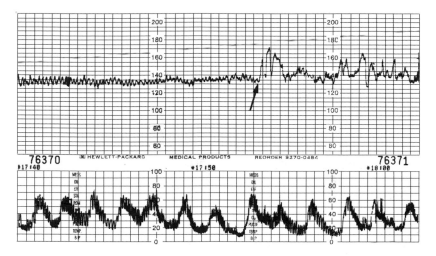

Figure 11.7 Sinusoidal-like trace: response to vibro-acoustic stimulus

have a stable baseline rate of 110–150 bpm with regular oscillations having an amplitude of 5–15 bpm (rarely greater), a frequency of 2–5 cycles per min and a fixed or flat baseline variability.[105] Usually the oscillations of the sinusoidal waveform above and below the baseline are equal. However, the most important feature is that there are no areas of normal FHR variability and there are no accelerations. Rhythmic fetal mouth movements (observed by ultrasound) in a healthy fetus have been associated with 'physiological' sinusoidal FHR patterns. When encountered with such a pattern, stimulation of the fetus (e.g. vibro-acoustic) should produce accelerations of the FHR (Fig. 11.7).[106] A fetus who is severely anaemic or hypoxic will not show accelerations, either spontaneously or in response to a stimulus (a child who is severely anaemic or hypoxic will not be able to throw a ball up and down and play). The neonatal outcome is the same in a fetus with spontaneous or sound-provoked accelerations observed on the FHR tracing. Reactivity and/or normal baseline variability in the FHR trace prior to or after the episode of a period of sinusoidal FHR pattern are suggestive of an uncompromised fetus. A 'saw-tooth' pattern of baseline variability instead of a smooth rounded sinusoidal waveform might suggest it is not a 'pathological' sinusoidal FHR pattern. Figures 11.8 and 11.9 show typical sinusoidal FHR patterns, one in a fetus with a haemoglobin of 3 g/dl (0.47 mmol/l) due to Rhesus disease. When such a trace is encountered the possibility of Rhesus disease, anaemia due to other causes like infection, haemoglobinopathies (Bart's thalassaemia), fetomaternal transfusion or bleeding from the fetus (vasa praevia) should be considered. Relevant investigations such as testing for Rhesus antibodies, the Kleihauer-Betke test to detect fetal cells in

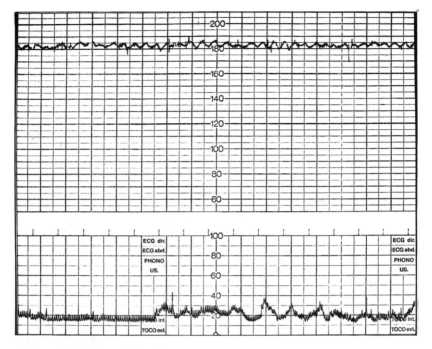

Figure 11.8 Sinusoidal pattern

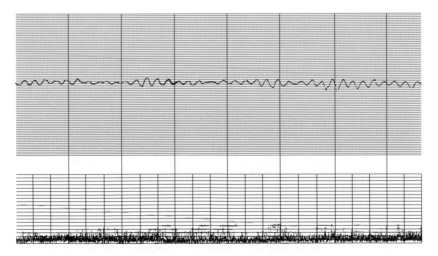

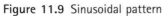

Figure 11.9 Sinusoidal pattern

the maternal blood, detection of thalassaemia carrier state or other appropriate investigations may be indicated.

At times sinusoidal heart rate patterns have been observed with the use of drugs like alphaprodine given to the mother.[107] Sometimes a typical sinusoidal pattern may not manifest and an atypical sinusoidal-like pattern may be seen in patients with fetal anaemia due to Rhesus disease or acute fetomaternal transfusion. Figure 11.10A shows a trace with most of the characteristics of sinusoidal pattern, but because of the absence of smooth sinus waveform and the unequal degree of oscillations above and below the baseline, the trace was not suspected to be abnormal and a decision was made not to consider this trace as sinusoidal in a growth-restricted fetus with no Rhesus disease. The trace was considered suspicious as there was no acceleratory response to sound. The non-stress test repeated three days later showed an ominous pattern (Fig. 11.10B). An immediate caesarean section was performed, and the baby had an Apgar score of 0, 0 and 3 at 1, 5 and 10 min respectively. The baby weighed 2.45 kg and had a haemoglobin level of 3.6 g/dl (0.56 mmol/l). The Kleihauer-Betke test on maternal blood was strongly positive, confirming a massive fetomaternal transfusion. The baby made a stormy recovery and subsequently developed cerebral palsy. 'Sinusoidal-like' traces are indicative of fetal anaemia[108,109] and can be recognized by familiarity with the typical pattern. Figure 11.11 shows another sinusoidal-like pattern due to fetomaternal transfusion.

Overdiagnosis of sinusoidal traces without applying proper criteria is associated with normal outcome. Sinusoidal traces may be atypical with a poor outcome. FBS in labour to determine fetal haemoglobin level and fetal blood gases can be useful.

FETAL BLEEDING

An antepartum haemorrhage may rarely be due to fetal bleeding. This is a serious threat to the fetus because of its limited circulating blood volume. A woman was admitted with a small antepartum haemorrhage and a surprising CTG (Fig. 11.12A). In most minor antepartum haemorrhages the CTG is normal because the bleeding is maternal blood and the placental circulation is not seriously threatened. In view of the CTG, induction of labour with continuous monitoring was undertaken. The CTG remained unusual (Fig. 11.12B) but, in the absence of decelerations, we were confident there was no progressive hypoxia. At 15.25 h there was a fresh vaginal bleed with a dramatic change in the CTG to a saltatory, pseudo-sinusoidal picture (Fig. 11.12C). This continued until delivery at 16.10 h (Fig. 11.12D). Delivery was by caesarean section when vasa praevia was noted and the baby was found to be anaemic. The baby made a good recovery after blood transfusion.

Dramatic changes in the CTG with minor antepartum haemorrhage suggest vasa praevia.

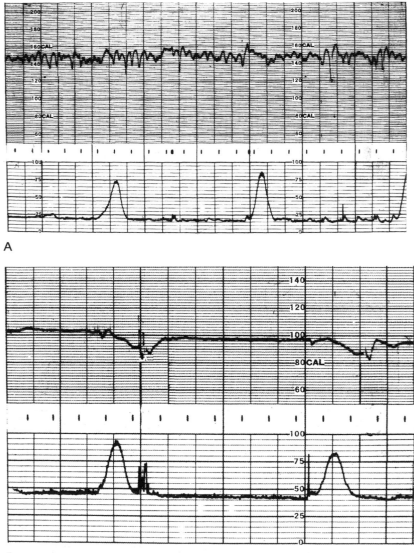

Figure 11.10 (A) Sinusoidal-like patterns: suspicious; (B) ominous

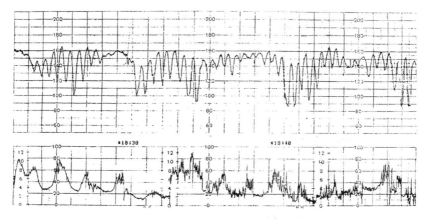

Figure 11.11 Sinusoidal-like pattern: fetomaternal transfusion

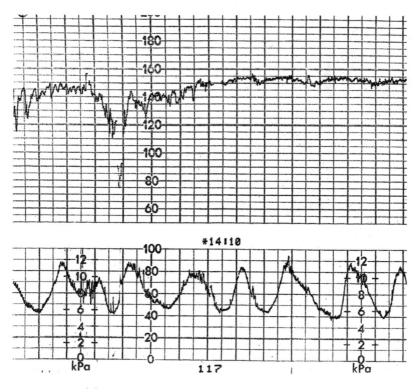

Figure 11.12 (A) CTG suscpicious therefore labour induced

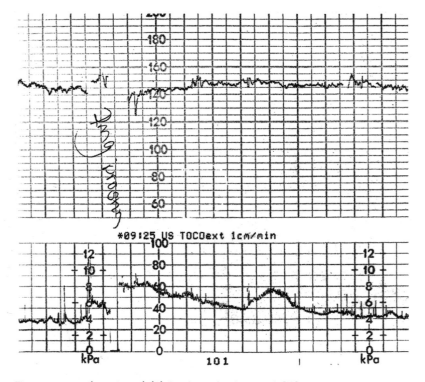

Figure 11.12 (*continued*) (B) Persistently abnormal CTG

THE DYING FETUS

Fetal death is always preceded by a terminal bradycardia. The trace preceding this may show a variety of features, most commonly a tachycardia.

Figure 11.13A–J shows 10 sequential hourly traces in a mismanaged case of a high-risk mother suffering from sickle-cell disease. This case occurred many years ago. The baby was known to be small with oligohydramnios. For reasons difficult to comprehend the medical staff failed to act and at delivery this baby was in serious trouble. Severe variable decelerations are seen with a classical progression to tachycardia, absence of accelerations, reduced variability and terminal bradycardia. The baby was a fresh stillbirth. Knowing that the patient was a high-risk nulliparous woman, all who have read this book would have delivered the baby by the time of the third strip of tracing, when the baby would have been in a reasonable condition. This high-risk woman had everything modern technology

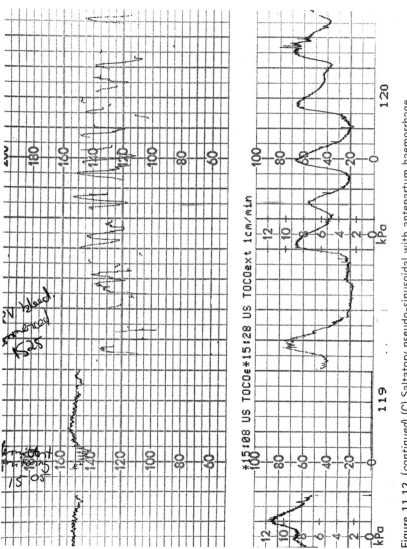

Figure 11.12 (*continued*) (C) Saltatory pseudo-sinusoidal with antepartum haemorrhage

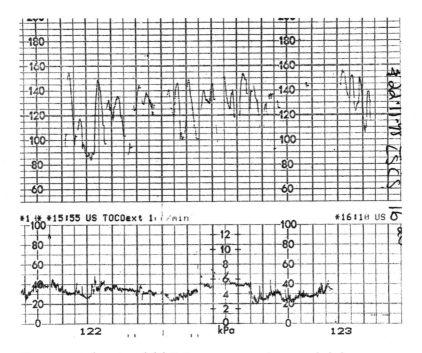

Figure 11.12 (*continued*) (D) Delivery vasa praevia, anaemic baby

could offer, with the notable exception of basic common sense on the part of the staff.

Some fetuses become so compromised in a more chronic way that they are unable to generate decelerations. This type of trace (Figs 11.14 and 11.15) is often misunderstood. There may be little in the way of a tachycardia but there is a complete absence of accelerations, a silent pattern of baseline variability and subtle, shallow late decelerations. This is an ominous picture and the baby must be delivered. These babies tend to have other clinical symptoms or signs such as absent fetal movements, intrauterine growth restriction, intrauterine infection, bleeding, post-term pregnancy or scanty fluid with thick meconium.

An ominous tracing demands delivery.

Birth asphyxia is often associated with prelabour asphyxia. This highlights the value of the admission test whenever there is a suspicion of fetal compromise or in an unbooked case. Should all babies with ominous traces be delivered with the expectation of a living, undamaged child? We are obliged to deliver all such babies but some features may indicate a poor prognosis.

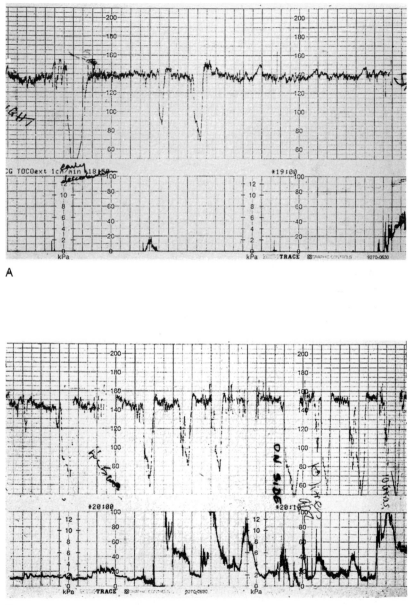

A

B

Figure 11.13 Dying fetus: (A) 1 h; (B) 2 h; (C) 3 h; (D) 4 h; (E) 5 h; (F) 6 h;
(G) 7 h; (H) 8 h; (I) 9 h; (J) 10 h

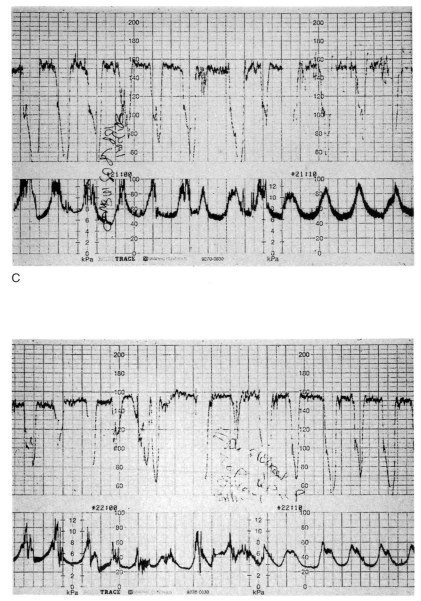

C

D

Figure 11.13 (continued)

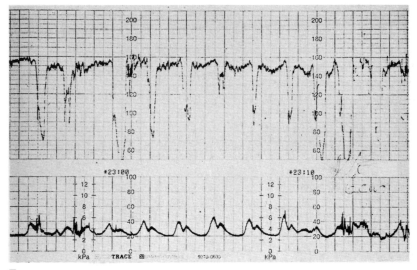

E

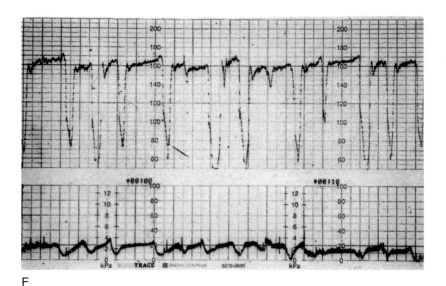

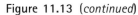

F

Figure 11.13 (*continued*)

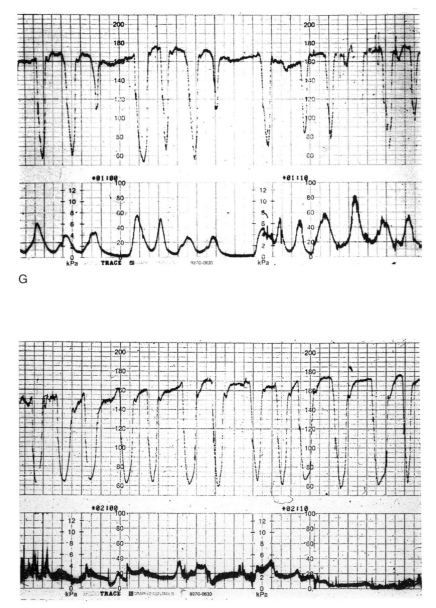

G

H

Figure 11.13 (*continued*)

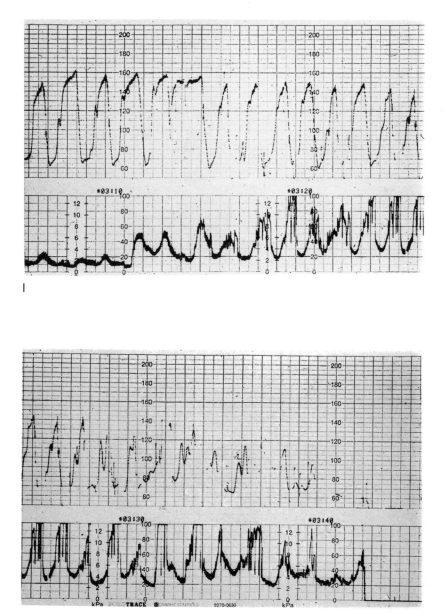

I

J

Figure 11.13 (continued)

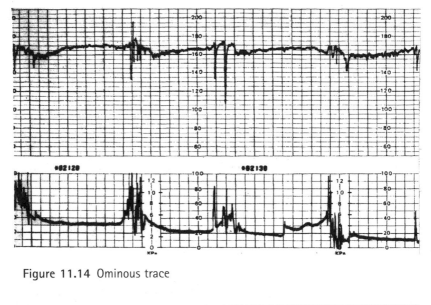

Figure 11.14 Ominous trace

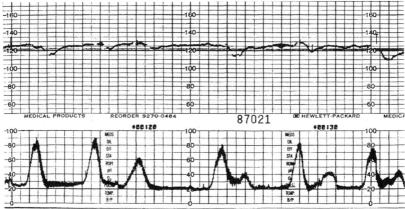
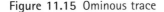

Figure 11.15 Ominous trace

A good trace within a reasonable period of the deterioration with an acute event such as an abruption suggests rapid intervention will be productive assuming a reasonable gestational age. Intervening when the main feature is tachycardia suggests some ability of the fetus to survive. Once the terminal bradycardia develops after the tachycardia the situation may be irretrievable (Fig. 11.16), especially when there are features of a random, uncontrolled undulatory pattern with no baseline variability (Fig. 11.17). This pattern suggests the possibility of central nervous system damage due to hypoxia. The

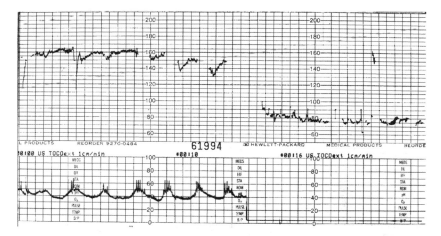

Figure 11.16 Terminal bradycardia

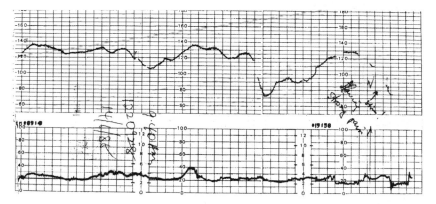

Figure 11.17 Terminal hypoxic central nervous system damage

challenge is to intervene in such pregnancies before this situation is reached; however, it should be kept in mind that central nervous system malformations can give rise to such patterns (see Ch. 6).

RECORDING OF THE MATERNAL HEART RATE THAT CAN MIMIC THE FETAL HEART RATE

Maternal heart rate (MHR) recording can mimic the FHR recording. This can arise in many situations and the steps to avoid this are:

1. Follow the current recommendation of the Medical Devices Agency. At the onset of the electronic fetal monitoring auscultate the FHR and apply the transducer, rather than cross-checking

with the maternal pulse. The reason for this is that the maternal pulse can be picked up by the ultrasound transducer and can be doubled (an increase of 100%), or it could be increased by 50%. It would be difficult to state whether the recording seen is that of the mother or the fetus.

2. It is also not uncommon for the machine to switch from fetal to maternal heart rate halfway through the recording. Any sudden shift in the baseline rate or a double baseline rate should indicate the possibility of recording the MHR and should warrant auscultation of the FHR.

3. Should there be a technically unsatisfactory recording with an ultrasound it is quite important that a scalp electrode is applied to obtain continuous FHR recording unless there is a contraindication to the use of fetal scalp electrode. This occurs more commonly in the late first and second stage of labour when the head moves down, or when the mother is restless, or there are too-frequent contractions with decelerations.

4. Be wary of a clear step change in the fetal heart pattern during the late first stage and the second stage of labour as the fetal head descends. This may not necessarily be a change in baseline rate, but rather a change in appearance (see Fig. 11.18). The overall features of baseline variability and reactivity seen on a trace are consistent throughout labour allowing for the normal variation of fetal sleep/wake cycles. At this stage of labour the baseline heart rates of mother and baby may be rather similar. The reappearance of accelerations is not reassuring after their preceding absence. It may be acceleration of the mother's heart (see below). Auscultation may help but application of a fetal scalp electrode will clarify the picture.

The following gives an explanation as to how these incidents occur. The characteristics of the MHR recording are different from that of the FHR recording in the second stage of labour. The FHR decelerates with head compression while the MHR increases with the uterine contractions. This should be identified and the FHR should be auscultated if there is any doubt. This knowledge should be disseminated widely to the maternity service practitioners (doctors and midwives). It would also be useful for those who are working in the community and midwifery birthing centres.

The appearance of the maternal heart rate in labour

The traces shown in Figure 5.25 are simultaneous recordings of the FHR (upper trace) and MHR (middle trace). The MHR is recorded by a precordial electrocardiograph (ECG) lead on the anterior aspect of the mother's chest and is indicated automatically by the machine as 'MECG' in between the contraction (lower trace) and the FHR chart channels. The MHR recording shows features of accelerations and increased baseline variability.

Unless closely observed for the accelerations corresponding to the contractions it is similar to the FHR. The MHR pattern in labour has been studied.[12] Following such studies the unintentional recording of MHR in labour has been increasingly reported[12,110] and it has been shown that increase of the MHR with contractions is present in most cases. *This rise in the baseline heart rate may be a response to the increased blood flowing into the maternal heart during the uterine contractions.* A typical example is shown in Figure 11.18.

The CTG shown in Figure 2.6 was that of a dead fetus and the signals were recorded with the use of a scalp electrode which shows the accelerations corresponding to the uterine contractions. In situations of fetal death the ultrasound transducer may pick up one of the maternal vessel pulsations and present it on the recorder, which gives a false impression of the FHR. If the characteristics of the MHR are not recognized one may continue to record, thinking that it is the FHR, only to find that the baby is stillborn or in a poor condition.

One has to think why the heart rate is accelerating with contractions in the late first and second stage of labour instead of having early or variable decelerations compatible with compression of the fetal head, as described in Chapter 8. Unfortunately this is not common knowledge to clinicians, nurses or midwives and many

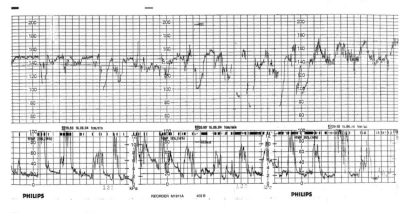

Figure 11.18 Observe the change in the fetal heart rate decelerative pattern with each contraction suddenly shifting to an accelerative pattern of maternal heart rate. The rise starts with the onset of the contractions and returns to its baseline rate with the offset of the contractions

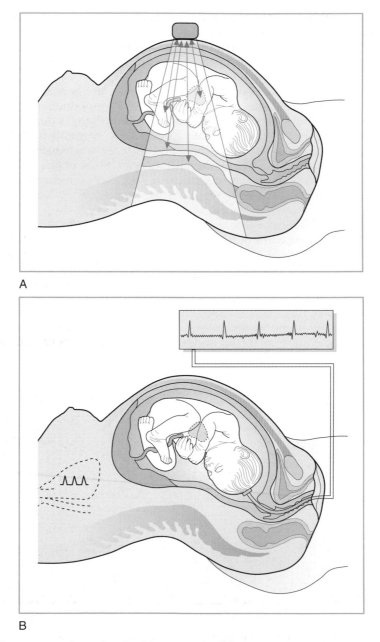

Figure 11.19 Recording fetal heart rate by (A) ultrasound transducer; (B) scalp electrode

interpret this as a FHR trace with accelerations in the second stage of labour. Alternatively they mistake the peak of the increase of the MHR to be the baseline FHR (if the MHR remains high for a longer duration) and the return of the MHR to its baseline rate as FHR decelerations.

Figure 11.19 illustrates how the fetal heart rate is recorded for continuous fetal heart rate monitoring. Mostly it is done using an ultrasound transducer or a scalp electrode. If the baby is dead there is a possibility that the maternal ECG could be transmitted via the electrode and recorded on the chart, and for observers to believe that it may be the FHR. Similarly the ultrasound transducer can pick up any pulsating maternal vessels, calculate the rate and record this on the chart, mimicking a FHR especially when there is no FHR or a very low FHR.

Figure 11.20 illustrates how the ultrasound transducer can slip from its original position where it was picking up the fetal heart, and then pick up a maternal pulsation, giving a trace of the MHR that may appear like the FHR, unless someone recognizes it and readjusts the transducer to get the FHR. If it was not recognized, the MHR would have been recorded without knowledge of the FHR until the end of labour. Here the sudden shift is obvious, but in exceptional cases it may be very subtle and difficult to pick up unless there is close scrutiny to observe the sudden changes in the baseline rate or the characteristics of the heart rate pattern.

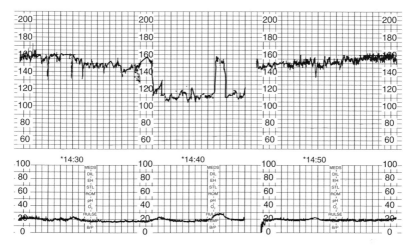

Figure 11.20 Recording by ultrasound – initial recording is that of the fetus. The ultrasound transducer slipped to the flank and picked up the maternal heart rate. This was identified and the transducer was replaced to record the fetal heart rate

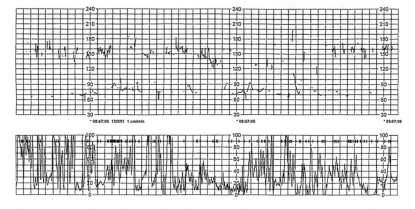

Figure 11.21 Trace showing fetal bradycardia of 70–75 bpm and doubling of the rate to 140 to 150 bpm thus giving two heart rates

It is known that the ultrasound transducer may pick up the maternal signal if the target signal moves away, such as after delivery of one twin or when there is sudden death of a fetus or acute fetal bradycardia.

Figure 11.21 shows how the machine doubles the FHR with bradycardia. In this case the two rates are seen, the lower line showing the true baseline FHR and the upper one the heart rate due to doubling. It is important to auscultate the FHR when two rates are recorded to identify whether it could be fetal or maternal.

At times the machine can record the MHR (perhaps doubled) with occasional glimpses of the FHR at a lower rate.[111] One should observe the heart rate in relation to the contractions with the bearing-down efforts in the second stage of labour. If the heart rate increases when the mother has painful contractions and returns to the baseline after the contraction returns to the baseline it is most likely to be the MHR because the FHR should decelerate with contractions due to head compression.

Chapter 12

The role of scalp pH

The availability of fetal scalp blood sampling for the assessment of fetal scalp capillary blood pH and its application in practice vary enormously. The NICE guidelines have suggested the use of scalp pH in situations with suspicious and/or pathological cardiotocography (CTG) after due consideration to the clinical situation.[13] At times the clinical situation may demand early delivery rather than a scalp pH. In reality, junior doctors use scalp pH more when they have less experience of labour ward responsibilities. This is understandable as they have a greater anxiety with a less-developed degree of understanding. As they gain experience and use pH as a guide, they then understand better the associations of an abnormal and a normal pH and will need this reassurance less often. The process of scalp blood sampling is undignified and uncomfortable for the woman. This is not to say it should not be done if properly indicated.

When the fetal heart rate (FHR) is reactive and normal, the chance of fetal acidosis is extremely low.[112–114] On the other hand, suspicious and abnormal FHR changes are not always associated with acidosis.[113–116] Such observations form the basis of the perceived need to measure fetal scalp pH for further investigation.

Changes in the CTG cause anxiety to the person not familiar with CTG interpretation. An inexperienced person in a centre with fetal blood sampling (FBS) facilities might perform FBS more frequently. When properly interpreted, assessment of FHR changes in most cases proves of equal value to pH in predicting fetal outcome.[14] FBS is a useful adjunct because, even with the worst pattern of tachycardia, reduced baseline variability and decelerations, only 50–60% of the fetuses are acidotic.[113] A wall chart correlating different FHR patterns to the percentage who are likely to be acidotic is available in most labour wards. It is clear from that chart and other studies that when the FHR pattern

exhibited accelerations the chance of fetal acidosis was zero, empha-
sizing accelerations as the hallmark of fetal health.[113] One problem
of these charts is that all fetuses do not conveniently provide a fetal
heart tracing that easily falls into one category. There is the added
perspective of the need for a time continuum, which is so important
in trace analysis.

Baseline variability is another good indicator of fetal health. When
normal baseline variability is observed in the last 20 min prior to
delivery, the babies are in good condition at birth regardless of other
features of the trace.[117] Fetal acidosis is more common when there is
a loss of baseline variability with tachycardia or late decelerations.[113,118] The preservation of normal baseline variability indicates
that the autonomic nervous system is responsive and the fetus is
trying to compensate despite other abnormal features in the trace.
The reason that, with a given FHR pattern, there are different per-
centages of fetuses showing acidosis depends on the duration for
which the suspicious or abnormal FHR pattern was present before
the time of FBS.[15] The approximate duration after which acidosis
develops in an appropriately grown term fetus with a given FHR
pattern has been discussed previously. It is also known that, in
fetuses with less 'placental reserve' such as those with intrauterine
growth restriction (IUGR), thick scanty meconium-stained fluid,[119]
in the presence of bleeding and in post-term infants, the rate of
decline of pH is steep compared with term infants appropriately
grown with abundant, clear amniotic fluid.

RESPIRATORY AND METABOLIC ACIDOSIS

Assessing pH alone does not suffice to identify the fetus at risk,
and more comprehensive blood gas analysis may be necessary for
clinical management. The placenta is the respiratory organ of the
fetus. Reduction of perfusion of the placenta from the fetal circulation
is manifest as variable decelerations due to cord compression, and
reduction of perfusion from the maternal circulation is manifest as
late decelerations. During the early stage of such threats the transfer
of carbon dioxide from the fetal to maternal side is reduced leading
to its accumulation. This results in respiratory acidosis manifested
by a low pH and a high PCO_2. Respiratory acidosis is transitory
particularly when corrective measures are taken and can be managed
conservatively provided the FHR pattern improves. With a further
reduction of perfusion from the maternal or fetal side the oxygen
transfer becomes affected leading to anaerobic metabolism and
metabolic acidosis in the fetus. This is manifested by a low pH,
low PO_2 and high base excess. Such metabolic acidosis is damaging
to the tissues. Transitory low pH values of respiratory type are

not uncommon in low-risk labours. Acidotic pH values in cord arterial blood in babies born with good Apgar scores are due to this phenomenon: 73% of babies with cord pH below 7.00 had a 1 min Apgar score of more than 7 and 86% had a 5 min Apgar score greater than 7.[120] These findings are probably due to respiratory acidosis which does not correlate well with fetal or neonatal condition. In this situation a comprehensive blood gas analysis, including PCO_2, base excess and preferably lactic acid, is desirable and more predictive. Caution should be exercised in using equipment that measures only pH. It is possible to determine the degree of metabolic acidosis by measuring the lactic acid level by the bedside with 5 µl of blood using the lactate card.[121] Intrauterine infection with a high metabolic rate presents a greater oxygen demand to the fetus and metabolic acidosis might develop with minimal interruption of placental perfusion.

WHEN TO DO FETAL BLOOD SAMPLING

Gradually developing hypoxia

The fetus becomes hypoxic and acidotic in labour in association with compromise of perfusion to the fetal or maternal side of the placental circulation. With the exception of situations of acute hypoxia due to cord prolapse, scar dehiscence, abruption and prolonged bradycardia, it is unusual for a fetus that has shown accelerations and good baseline variability to become hypoxic without developing decelerations in labour. The decelerations indicate the presence of stress to the fetus, whether from the challenge of poor perfusion or mechanical pressure. Provided the baseline FHR has not started to rise and there is no reduction in the baseline variability to less than 5 beats, there is little to be gained by performing FBS, as the pH is likely to be normal unless the decelerations are prolonged and last for a duration two to three times greater than the duration of baseline FHR between the decelerations. If the baseline FHR has risen by 20–30 beats and is not showing any further rise, with a reduction in variability to less than 5 beats, then distress is probable. Despite the fetus having increased its cardiac output to a possible maximum by increasing the FHR, the functioning of the autonomic nervous system controlling the baseline variability is compromised by hypoxia. The time course of this process may be referred to as the *stress-to-distress period*. This period varies from fetus to fetus depending on the physiological reserve. This reserve is critically low in high-risk situations of postmaturity, IUGR, intrauterine infection and in those with thick meconium and scanty amniotic fluid.

When the FHR shows hypoxic features suggestive of distress it is important to perform an FBS for pH and blood gases as the fetus may be, or become, acidotic. Initially this will be a respiratory, followed by metabolic, acidosis. Once the FHR shows a distress pattern (markedly reduced baseline variability with late or atypical variable decelerations), the time taken for metabolic acidosis to develop is unpredictable. This pattern is referred to as *preterminal pattern* by some authors. After a certain duration of the distress pattern (the distress period) the FHR starts to decline in a rapid stepwise pattern, culminating in terminal bradycardia and death (the distress-to-death period). The stress-to-distress interval (20.00 h–00.00 h, i.e. 4 h), the distress period (00.00 h–03.00 h, i.e. 3 h) and the distress-to-death period (03.00 h–03.40 h, i.e. 40 min) are illustrated by Figure 11.13A–J. Another example where the stress-to-distress period, the distress period and the distress-to-death period are much shorter is shown in Figure 7.4A–F. Clinical interpretation of the FHR pattern will identify the onset of stress, distress and the stress-to-distress period. It will also identify the fetus in the distress period. An accurate prediction of the distress period cannot be made based on the FHR pattern as illustrated by these two examples. During the final decline phase (distress-to-death period), when the fetal heart rate drops irretrievably within a short period, it is often too late to intervene.

The value of FBS may be at the onset of the distress period and again repeated 30–40 min later or earlier, depending on the first pH and base excess, baseline variability and the type of decelerations. Adherence to the recommendation of immediate delivery when the pH is less than 7.20 (acidosis), and a repeat sample in 30 min or less when the pH was 7.20–7.25 (pre-acidosis) is good practice. Previous recommendations were that when the pH was greater than 7.25 repeat sampling was not required unless the FHR deteriorated. This approach may generate a false sense of security when the trace does not deteriorate, although the pH is declining. Repeat measurement in appropriate time based on the first pH, and the abnormality of the trace even when the first pH is in the normal range, helps to identify the rate of decline.[122] A decision for delivery can be made considering the rate of decline of the pH, the clinical risk factors (IUGR, thick meconium), parity, current cervical dilatation and rate of progress of labour.

Subacute hypoxia

The pH may deteriorate rapidly in a fetus who previously had a reactive trace without an increase in the baseline FHR, if the decelerations are pronounced with large dip areas (drop of more than 60 beats per min (bpm) for over 90 s) with the FHR recovering to the baseline only for short periods of time (less than 60 s). Examples of such traces are shown in Figure 12.1A–F. In these situations a drop in pH can be by as much as 0.01 every 3–4 min. This decline in pH will be even steeper if the preceding trace was suspicious or abnormal or the clinical picture was one of high risk (IUGR, thick meconium with scanty fluid, or intrauterine infection). Further insults at this time, such as oxytocin infusion or a difficult instrumental delivery, may make the situation worse. With such traces, attempts at FBS will delay much-needed urgent delivery.

Chronic hypoxia

A non-reactive FHR pattern showing a baseline variability less than 5 beats with shallow decelerations (less than 15 beats for 15 s), even with a normal baseline rate, indicates severe compromise and delivery should be expedited without delay to avoid fetal death (see Fig. 7.6A–D). A non-reactive trace with a baseline variability of less than 5 beats but without decelerations lasting more than 90 min indicates the possibility of already existing hypoxic compromise or damage due to other reasons (e.g. cerebral haemorrhage). This needs further evaluation if the pH is normal. In these circumstances fetal death may occur suddenly without further warning of a rise in baseline FHR or decelerations (see Fig. 7.5A–J). Hence, a non-reactive trace for greater than 90 min is abnormal and is an indication for further evaluation to rule out hypoxia.

Acute hypoxia

Abruption, cord prolapse, scar dehiscence and uterine hyperstimulation may give rise to acute hypoxia. This may manifest as prolonged bradycardia; at other times prolonged bradycardia occurs without obvious reason and in all circumstances is associated with rapidly progressive acidosis. With a bradycardia of less than 80 bpm the pH is likely to decline at the rate of approximately 0.01 per min.[87] The decline may be steeper in the presence of an abnormal trace prior to the bradycardia.

With FHR patterns suggestive of acute or subacute hypoxia, performing a FBS might delay intevention, resulting in poor outcome. In FHR patterns with poor variability lasting for more than 90 min, but with no decelerations, investigations should be performed to identify the cause. The principle can be established that the FHR pattern identifies the onset of stress (decelerations) and of distress (maximal elevation of baseline FHR with baseline variability less than 5 beats). Although the onset of stress and distress can be identified, the duration of the distress period before the fetus becomes hypoxic

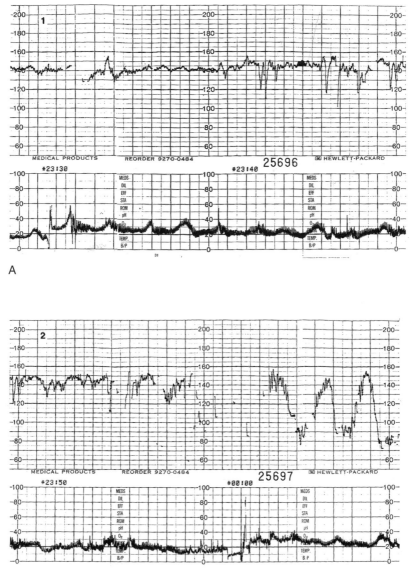

A

B

Figure 12.1 (A–F) Subacute hypoxia: prolonged decelerations (>90 s, depth >60 bpm) with short intervals of recovery (<60 s) to baseline rate

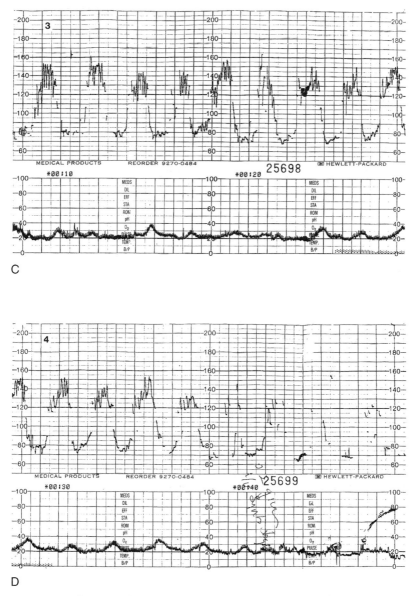

C

D

Figure 12.1 (*continued*)

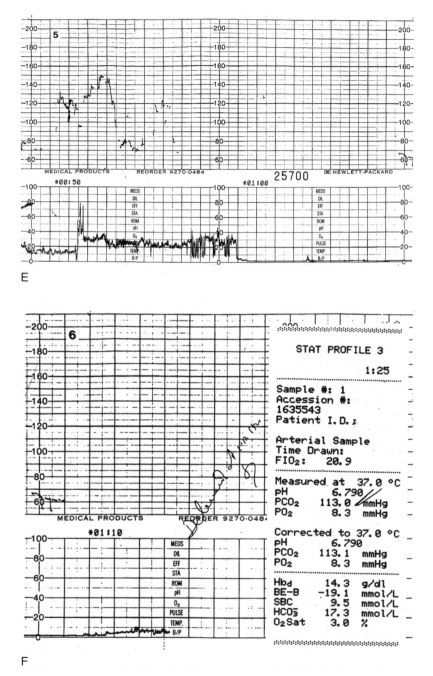

E

F

Figure 12.1 (continued)

and acidotic cannot be predicted. A decision is required to deliver or to perform FBS, bearing in mind the clinical picture, if the prospect of early delivery is poor.

Alternative methods like electrocardiograph waveform analysis and pulse oximetry are being used as adjuncts to CTG for monitoring the fetus. They have a place only in assisting clinical decision making when the FHR starts to become suspicious, and should be used only after acquiring adequate knowledge and training of how to use them. They are useful adjuncts and may replace FBS. Computer-assisted interpretation of the CTG is likely to assist in decision making especially in judging baseline variability when the CTG becomes suspicious or abnormal. When the CTG is normal there is no need for the adjunctive methods.

WHEN NOT TO DO FETAL BLOOD SAMPLING

Frequently the FHR changes observed might be due to factors other than hypoxia. Dehydration, ketosis, maternal pyrexia and anxiety can give rise to fetal tachycardia but do not usually present with decelerations. Occipitoposterior position is known to be associated with more variable decelerations without hypoxic features, evidenced by normal baseline rate and variability.[123] Oxytocin can cause hyperstimulation resulting in FHR changes of various forms, which have been discussed in an earlier chapter. Prolonged bradycardia can be due to postural hypotension following epidural analgesia. FHR changes should be correlated with the clinical picture before action is taken. In many instances remedial action such as hydration, repositioning of the mother or stopping the oxytocin infusion will relieve the FHR changes and no further action is necessary. When the FHR changes persist despite such actions, a FBS or one of the stimulation tests is warranted. At times FBS may not be necessary because the trace is reassuring with accelerations and normal baseline variability despite some decelerations (Fig. 12.4), or it may show a low result transiently and later show a good result; the pH may be low transiently due to respiratory acidosis. Above all, when the trace is ominous or the clinical picture is poor it is better to deliver the baby rather than wasting time with FBS. At times a false reassurance leads to an unsatisfactory outcome.

Scalp FBS is often not appropriate under the following circumstances:

1. When the clinical picture demands early delivery (Fig. 12.2): 42 weeks' gestation, cervix 3 cm dilated, thick meconium with scanty fluid

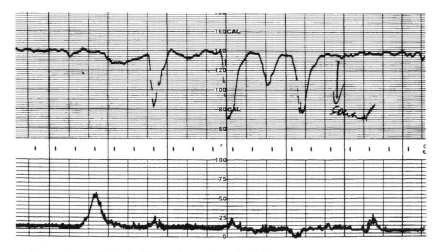

Figure 12.2 Clinical picture demands early delivery

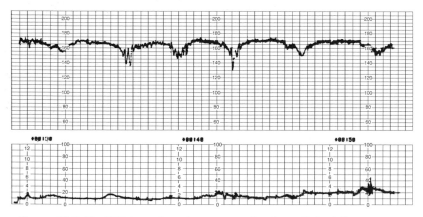

Figure 12.3 The FHR trace is ominous prompting immediate delivery

2. When an ominous trace prompts immediate delivery (Fig. 12.3)
3. When the FHR trace is reassuring (Fig. 12.4)
4. When the changes are due to oxytocic overstimulation (see Fig. 10.5)
5. When there is associated persistent failure to progress in labour (Fig. 12.5)
6. During, or soon after, an episode of prolonged bradycardia (see Fig. 10.4)

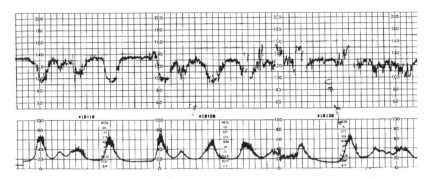

Figure 12.4 FHR in the second stage – reassuring

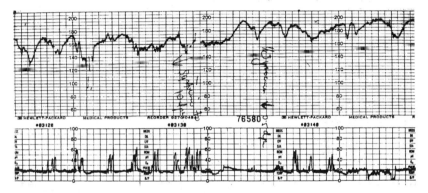

Figure 12.5 Changes in FHR: failure to progress in labour

7. If spontaneous vaginal delivery is imminent or easy instrumental vaginal delivery is possible (see Fig. 8.15).

Following these principles will help to avoid unnecessary FBS, operative deliveries and fetal morbidity from undue delay in delivery.

ALTERNATIVES TO FETAL BLOOD SAMPLING

In practice FBS may not be performed because the facilities or the expertise are not available, or because it is technically difficult. Alternative indirect methods are useful in this situation. A retrospective observation and correlation of the scalp blood pH to the presence or absence of accelerations at the time of FBS (Fig. 12.6) led to the *scalp stimulation test*.[124] When the scalp was stimulated by

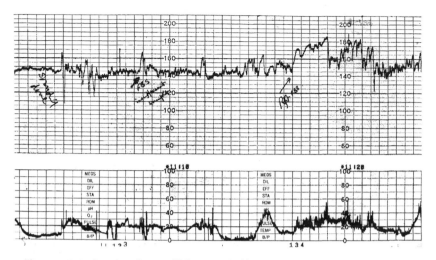

Figure 12.6 Acceleration at FBS, normal pH

Table 12.1 Results of scalp stimulation tests in relation to scalp blood pH values[124–126]

Response to scalp stimulation	Fetal scalp blood pH values			
	<7.20 (n = 82)	7.20–7.25 (n = 156)	>7.25 (n = 462)	Total (n = 700)
POSITIVE RESPONSE	1 (0.4%)	33 (12.7%)	226 (86.9%)	260
NEGATIVE RESPONSE	40 (44.4%)	45 (50.0%)	5 (5.6%)	90
TOTAL	41 (11.7%)	78 (22.3%)	231 (66%)	350

pinching with a tissue forceps, if an acceleration was present it was unlikely that the scalp blood pH was below 7.20.[125,126] On the other hand, if there were no accelerations to such a stimulus only about 50% had acidotic pH values (<7.20), whereas a significant proportion had pre-acidotic values (7.20–7.25) and others had normal values (Table 12.1).

Therefore this test was useful in identifying those who are not at risk, although it was not good in predicting those who are likely to be acidotic. In centres where facilities do not exist for scalp FBS, such a test would be a useful adjunct in reducing the number of unnecessary caesarean sections for 'fetal distress', and in centres where facilities are available for FBS, it will reduce the number of samples taken. Where there is a failure to obtain a sample during the FBS procedure, observation of an acceleration is very reassuring and the procedure can be discontinued.

In the study described above, the case that recorded a positive response with an acidotic pH (see Table 12.1) showed respiratory acidosis, which is due to accumulation of CO_2, is not harmful to the fetus and is known to reverse itself once the FHR returns to normal. Careful observation of the characteristics of the FHR resulted in a fetus born with good Apgar scores.

An alternative to the scalp stimulation test is a *fetal acoustic stimulation test* (FAST) in labour (Fig. 12.7).[127] There were a number of reports from the USA showing the fetus responding with FHR acceleration to FAST if it was not acidotic. Although the majority of fetuses with non-acidotic pH responded with accelerations, when they failed to respond only about 50% had acidotic pH values, which was similar to the results of the scalp stimulation test. It is difficult to explain why the fetal response of accelerations should be associated with arbitrary cut-off points of scalp blood pH values; however, it is known that auditory sensation is one of the first to be affected by hypoxia and negative response to acoustic stimulation might warn of the possibility of hypoxia. Fetal acoustic stimulation is a new modality used to test fetal wellbeing and concern has been raised about safety aspects. Studies performed on its safety have shown that there is no evidence of catecholamine release with the stimulus,[128] no hearing loss[129] and

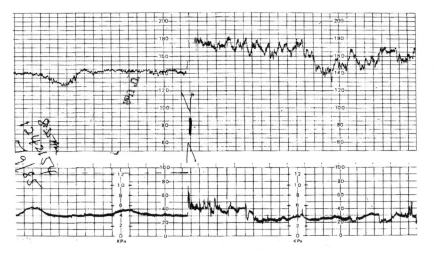

Figure 12.7 Accelerative response to vibro-acoustic stimulus

no long-term disturbance to the fetal behavioural state studied by FHR variability cycles.[130] With these alternative methods available there is a tendency for physicians to perform FBS less frequently, and even a willingness to replace this test by FAST or scalp stimulation tests.[131] Care should be exercised if relying on such stimulation tests alone, because 50% of fetuses who do not show a reaction to the FAST or scalp stimulation have non-acidotic pH values; and some fetuses show a positive response even with acidotic pH values due to respiratory acidosis (Fig. 12.8).[132,133]

The Royal College of Obstetricians and Gynaecologists Study Group and NICE have recommended that fetal scalp blood sampling facilities should be available in any hospital where electronic fetal monitoring is performed.[134] However, clinicians who understand the clinical situation and the FHR pattern may make a decision without resorting to FBS and without an increase in caesarean section rate for fetal distress.[131] In many situations it may be wiser to proceed to delivery without wasting precious time. It has been shown that if the decision-to-delivery interval in situations of fetal distress is 35 min as opposed to 15 min the admission rate to the neonatal intensive care unit is doubled.[135] FBS is not always possible because facilities may not be available or it may be difficult to perform due to an undilated cervix or high head.[136,137] In these situations, decisions based on the CTG and the clinical situation remain critical.

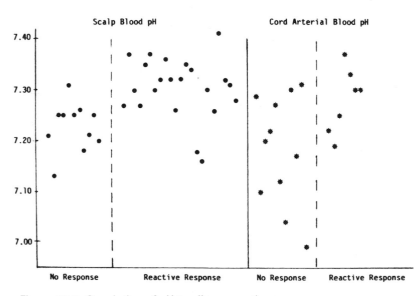

Figure 12.8 Correlation of pH to vibro-acoustic response

POINTS TO PONDER

Although pH is a useful adjunct, the following points should be considered in clinical decision making:[133]

- Accelerations and normal baseline variability are hallmarks of fetal health.
- Accelerations without baseline variability should be considered suspicious.
- Periods of decreased baseline variability without decelerations may represent quiet fetal sleep.
- Hypoxic fetuses may have a normal baseline FHR of 110–160 bpm with no accelerations and baseline variability <5 bpm for >40 mins (in the absence of adverse clinical parameters, observation for >90 mins may be needed to recognize the abnormality).
- In the presence of baseline variability of <5 bpm, even shallow decelerations of <15 bpm are ominous in a non-reactive trace.
- Abruption, cord prolapse and scar rupture can cause acute hypoxia and should be suspected clinically (may give rise to prolonged decelerations/bradycardia).
- Fetal hypoxia and acidosis may develop faster with an abnormal trace when there is scanty, thick meconium, IUGR, intrauterine infection with pyrexia and/or pre- or post-term labour.
- In preterm fetuses (especially <34 weeks), hypoxia and acidosis can increase the likelihood of respiratory distress syndrome and may contribute to intraventricular haemorrhage, warranting early intervention in the presence of an abnormal trace.
- Hypoxia can be made worse by injudicious use of oxytocin, epidural analgesia and difficult operative deliveries.
- During labour, if decelerations are absent, asphyxia is unlikely although it cannot be completely excluded.
- Abnormal patterns may represent the effects of drugs, fetal anomaly, fetal injury or infection – not only hypoxia.

Chapter 13

Alternative methods of intrapartum fetal surveillance

Despite the limited contribution of birth asphyxia to cerebral palsy and doubts cast on the benefits of intrapartum electronic fetal monitoring, research is in progress to find better methods of monitoring to avoid the tragedies which can occur due to birth asphyxia. Every now and then such tragedies are highlighted by litigation and the large awards of damages. There is little doubt that the practice of intrapartum fetal monitoring is likely to stay, but whether it will be in the form of electronic fetal heart rate (FHR) monitoring or by other means, or a by a combination, is difficult to predict. This chapter reviews why there is a search for newer methods, some of the newer methods available and what may happen in the future.

WHY IS THERE A SEARCH FOR NEW METHODS?

There are problems in correlating FHR changes with fetal acidosis. When all four features of the cardiotocograph (CTG) trace are normal, the chances of fetal acidosis are small. When all the features are abnormal just over 50% are noted to be acidotic.[113] Depending on the physiological reserve of each fetus, one may respond differently from another to the hypoxic insult. It has been observed that for 50% of appropriately grown term fetuses with clear amniotic fluid to get acidotic, it takes 115 min with repetitive late decelerations, 145 min with repetitive variable decelerations and 185 min with a 'flat trace' (i.e. with reduced baseline variability).[15] This implies that some appropriately grown term fetuses may become acidotic in a shorter period. This duration may be even shorter when there is reduced physiological reserve, i.e. in cases with infection, bleeding, post-term, growth-restriction and in those with scanty, thick, meconium-stained fluid. Therefore, it becomes necessary to determine the fetal condition when there are abnormal FHR changes by fetal scalp blood sampling (FBS). This will help to identify those in need of delivery and to avoid unnecessary operative intervention. However, the facilities and expertise are not available to perform FBS in many centres,[136,137] and its value is questioned by some.[131] It is also known that FBS is done when it is not warranted and is not done when it is needed.[138] In addition, the intermittent nature of the readings also makes it difficult to identify the optimal time to intervene without compromising the fetus, without increasing operative interventions. These issues have prompted research into newer methods of fetal surveillance in labour which are used as adjuncts to CTG in some centres.

FETAL ELECTROCARDIOGRAPH WAVEFORM ANALYSIS

The concept of electrocardiograph (ECG) waveform analysis relies on changes in the ST segment of the fetal ECG. They are related to metabolic events in the fetal myocardium during hypoxia. The changes in time constants, like the PR or RR intervals (FHR), were tried to identify cases of acidosis but the methodology has not advanced for it to be used in clinical practice. On the basis of experimental data, together with developments in bioengineering, advances have been made in the computerized analysis of ST waveform in the last few years. The STAN-ST analyser (Neoventa, Gotenborg, Sweden) is a CTG machine which gives a CTG trace, and when the CTG is obtained using a scalp electrode in labour it analyses the ST waveform.

Experimental data have suggested that the appearance of high-peaked T waves together with an elevation of the ST segment signifies an imbalance of the myocardial energy situation with anaerobic metabolism and myocardial glycogenolysis. This important defence mechanism is known to operate with an increase in circulating catecholamine (β-adrenoceptor stimulation):[139] this brings about a shift in K^+ which increases the T-wave amplitude (T/QRS ratio) (Fig. 13.1A and B). The detection of ST changes are computerized and the STAN equipment highlights any significant changes in the ST segment. The ST events detected may be a *baseline rise* of the T/QRS ratio, an *episodic rise* of the T/QRS ratio or a *biphasic ST* segment. Each fetus has a steady level of T/QRS ratio in early labour that could be identified from the initial recording. The rise in the T/QRS ratio is calculated in reference to the lowest T/QRS ratio calculated over a period of 20 min in the previous 3 h period. This means that the equipment needs to be used for 20 min to calculate the baseline T/QRS ratio prior to major changes in heart rate or the ECG. In the immediate 20 min after start up, and when there are poor discontinuous signals, manual data analysis is required. A *preterminal trace*

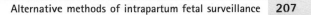

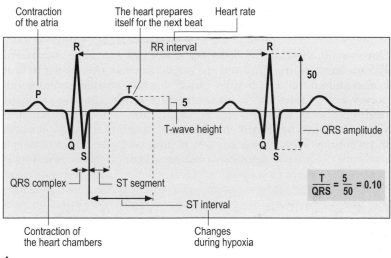

A

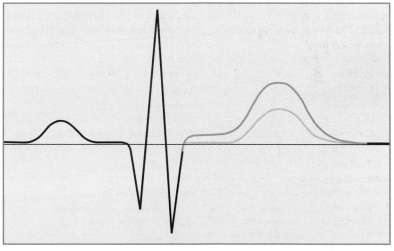

B

Figure 13.1 (A) Measurement of T/QRS ratio; (B) ST elevation and rise in the T wave

that shows total lack of baseline variability and reactivity, with or without decelerations, and a prolonged deceleration warrant immediate delivery.

A steadily increasing T/QRS rise is termed a *baseline rise*, and if the ratio increases significantly and comes down within a brief period of a few minutes it is termed an *episodic rise*. The biphasic event refers to alteration of the ST segment where there is an initial rise and then a fall (Fig. 13.2). If the ST change is above the isoelectric line, it is termed biphasic 1; if it cuts the isoelectric line it is called biphasic 2; and if it is below the isoelectric line it is called biphasic 3. Biphasic 2 and 3 are considered significant and are related to the electrical flow from endocardium to epicardium. Hence these changes may present themselves in the following situations: when the myocardium is thin (e.g. preterm fetuses), there is myocardial disease, infection and hypoxia.[140]

The FHR pattern, the ECG complex with T/QRS analysis, and uterine contractions are recorded online on the same trace as shown in Figure 13.3.

The changes in the T/QRS ratio are highlighted as STAN events on the CTG trace if they are significant, and are recorded on a log event on the screen. The early studies in the 1980s showed promising results,[141,142] but inconsistent results from other studies[143] highlighted

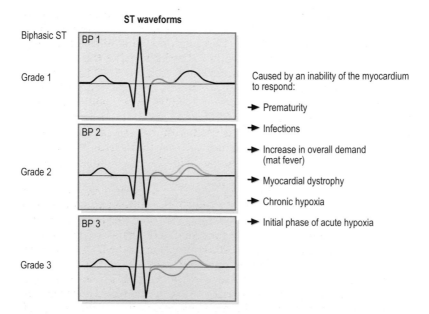

Figure 13.2 The different grades of biphasic events

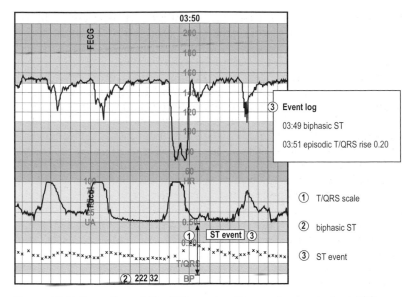

Figure 13.3 Recording of the FHR, contractions and computerized ECG waveform analysis of T/QRS plotted on the lower channel of the trace

the need for computerization of ECG analysis and to take a rise in T/QRS from its own baseline levels instead of considering fixed values applicable to all fetuses. Two randomized studies, consisting of nearly 4500 subjects, based on an algorithm using the combined analysis of CTG and ECG waveform analysis (Table 13.1) have shown a reduction in the caesarean section rate and the incidence of metabolic acidosis when the ECG waveform analysis was used in conjunction with CTG, compared with CTG alone (Table 13.2).[144,145]

The ECG waveform analysis is used with the CTG, as STAN or ST events can present due to mechanical stresses to the fetus. In addition to the above decision algorithm, the following guidelines apply for using the STAN technology.

This technology is applicable to pregnancies that are 36 weeks complete or more. Significant ST events, when judged along with the CTG, indicate the need for intervention. This could be delivery of the fetus or alleviation of a cause of abnormal FHR changes such as oxytocin overstimulation or maternal hypotension. If the ST event takes place in the active second stage of labour, immediate delivery is recommended. If the CTG is suspicious or abnormal in the second stage and if the ST analyser was started when the CTG was normal, or immediately after the trace became suspicious in the first stage of labour, then one could wait for 90 min before intervention.

Table 13.1 Decision-making algorithm using computerized analysis of ECG waveform with visual interpretation of the CTG

ST analysis	Intermediary CTG	Abnormal CTG	Preterminal CTG
Episodic T/QRS rise	>0.15	>0.10	Immediate
Baseline T/QRS rise	>0.10	>0.05	Delivery
Biphasic ST	Continuous >5 min or >2 episodes of coupled biphasic 2 or biphasic 3	Continuous >2 min or >1 episode of coupled biphasic 2 or biphasic 3	

Table 13.2 The results of the Plymouth and Swedish randomized studies that show reduction in operative delivery rates for fetal distress and the incidence of metabolic acidosis at delivery[144,145]

	Plymouth RCT[144]	Swedish RCT[145]
Operative delivery for fetal distress		
Control arm	9.1%	9.3%
STAN arm	5.0%	7.7%
Metabolic acidosis		
Control arm	1.40%	1.44%
STAN arm	0.55%	0.57%

When a STAN event is flagged up by the STAN equipment, one has to note the type of STAN event and the magnitude of change in that event, e.g. a baseline T/QRS rise of 0.06 or episodic T/QRS rise of 0.09. Having noted this, one has to interpret the CTG as abnormal or suspicious to decide on the action to be taken. If the CTG is pathological then action is warranted with a baseline rise of 0.06 or an episodic rise >0.10. The CTG classification used in the Swedish study[145] is slightly different from the NICE guidelines.[13]

A baseline rate of 110–150 bpm was considered normal, early and simple variable decelerations <60 beats and <60 s were considered normal, and variable decelerations <60 s but with beat loss >60 beats were considered suspicious in the Swedish study.[145]

The case shown in Figures 13.4–13.6 illustrates the use of the STAN technology. A primigravid needed augmentation for poor progress

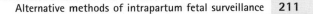
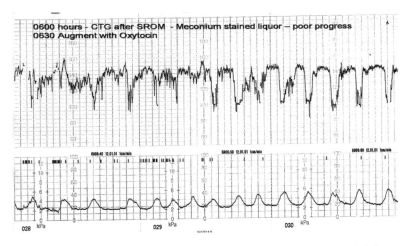

Figure 13.4 Cardiotocograph showing variable decelerations in early labour – related to hyperstimulation with oxytocin used for augmentation of labour

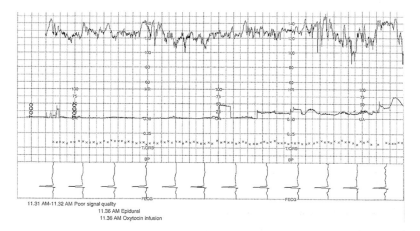

Figure 13.5 Oxytocin infusion was stopped. The cardiotocograph returned to normal and was reactive with no decelerations, but the contractions became less frequent. The ST analyser was connected and oxytocin infusion restarted

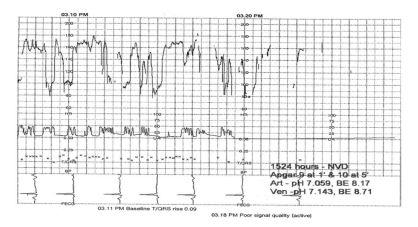

Figure 13.6 There was a gradual rise in the baseline rate following decelerations, followed by reduction in baseline variability. No fetal blood sampling was done as there were no ST events. At 15.11 h there was an ST event of baseline rise indicating the need for delivery. A spontaneous delivery was imminent and the woman delivered spontaneously at 15.24 h. The baby had good Apgar scores and no evidence of metabolic acidosis

of labour. Variable decelerations are seen with oxytocin hyperstimulation. When oxytocin was stopped or reduced the contractions became less frequent, lasting for a shorter duration and no progress was being made. The ST analyser was used for continuous additional information. Even if the fetus showed FHR decelerations and an increase in baseline rate, the absence of STAN events (significant ECG changes) would give reassurance to continue with the oxytocin infusion with the aim of achieving a normal vaginal delivery.

SYSTOLIC TIME INTERVALS OF THE FETAL CARDIAC CYCLE

Laboratory and clinical studies have suggested that the systolic time intervals (STIs) of the cardiac cycle may be sensitive indicators of cardiac function and fetal compromise. The main STIs are the pre-ejection period (PEP) from the onset of ventricular depolarization to the opening of the aortic valve, and the ventricular ejection time (VET) from the aortic opening to aortic closure. The PEP is an indicator of myocardial contractility and the VET mainly reflects peripheral resistance.

The QRS complex of the fetal heart, derived in labour by scalp electrode, provides an easily obtainable and identifiable signal of ventricular polarization. The precise and consistent identification of aortic valvular events is difficult. The most satisfactory available technique relies on Doppler ultrasound for the detection of cardiac motion. The detection of individual valvular events is effected by a series of time and amplitude gates. The signals that pass through these gates are regenerated to provide precise indications of the timing of mitral valve closure, aortic valve opening and closure, and mitral valve opening. Similar signals are derived from the fetal electrocardiogram. From these signals, the intervals can be determined electronically. The digital measurements of time can then be converted to analogue form for recording alongside uterine activity and FHR on a strip chart recorder. In pregnancy, STIs are affected by many factors besides myocardial compromise, including heart rate, gestational age, birth weight, cardiac preload and afterload, hypoxia and acidosis.[146] From animal and human adult studies it is known that STIs can also be affected by peripheral resistance, inotropic drugs, valvular disease and cardiac arrhythmias.[147] Fetal STIs have been studied for changes associated with FHR patterns during labour. Periodic accelerations are associated with prolongation of PEP and shortening of VET. Early decelerations are associated with a mild prolongation of periodic PEP,[148] and a slight prolongation of VET, inversely proportional to the FHR.[149] Variable decelerations are associated with prolonged periodic PEP values. Changes in VET are variable and prolonged VETs were seen with severe decelerations because of the inverse relationship with FHR. The relationship between STI changes and late decelerations is not clear and is probably dependent on whether fetal hypoxia is acute or chronic, and the presence of acidosis. It is likely that shortening of baseline PEP occurs with late decelerations in early stages, while prolongation of PEP, reflecting myocardial depression, occurs with severe (hypoxic) late decelerations and acidosis. During labour, STIs may prove to be of value in elucidating equivocal FHR patterns, and in detecting fetal hypoxia and acidosis. A shortening of the baseline PEP between contractions may reflect the onset and progression of hypoxia. However, technical improvements are required together with further clinical studies comparing STI measurements with current monitoring techniques to define the sensitivity and specificity.

PULSE OXIMETRY

Modern monitoring of anaesthetic and neonatal patients includes pulse oximetry. Pulse oximeters are cheap and non-invasive, and monitor both heart rate and arterial oxygen saturation (SaO_2). The accuracy of the method has been established and, unlike partial pressure of oxygen (PaO_2) monitors, pulse oximeters respond rapidly to changes in the oxygen content in the blood.

There are specific advantages of recording SaO_2 instead of PaO_2. The oxygen pressure electrode requires frequent calibration, and necessitates shaving hair and firm fixation techniques. The relation of oxygen saturation and partial pressure is defined by the oxygen dissociation curve, and a small change in PaO_2 is represented by a large change in SaO_2; large changes are easier to detect and are less affected by technical errors. An increase in hydrogen ion concentration or 2,3-diphosphoglycerate shifts the oxygen dissociation curve to the right: a baby who is acutely or chronically hypoxaemic and/or acidaemic may have a normal PaO_2 but its oxygen saturation will be low. However, obvious disadvantages exist with the use of pulse oximetry in labour: the cervix must be open enough to insert the probe. There are oximetry probes and equipment available to measure oxygen saturation with intact membranes. Several studies of the use of pulse oximetry in labour have been conducted.[150–154] Most published studies are with sensors that are in contact with the fetal cheek. The new sensors that are incorporated with a scalp electrode show promise, but studies from different centres are needed to test the efficacy of these electrodes in producing continuous signals. Oxygen saturation readings have been shown not to be affected in fetuses with meconium staining of the amniotic fluid.

The deoxygenated blood in the inferior vena cava of the fetus mixes with oxygenated blood from the umbilical vein and, hence, scalp oximetry readings are less than the values found in the umbilical vein. The readings tend to range from 30–80% and, in the same fetus, the values can fluctuate widely at different dilatations without hypoxia or acidosis.[152] The details of the basic principles, technology and clinical issues of pulse oximetry are discussed elsewhere.[155,156]

One particular sensor (Nellcor®), which is wedged between the cheek and the uterus, has been used for most studies, and successful readings have been obtained in 65–85% of cases in labour.[152,157] Pulse oximetry has also been used in conjunction with CTG. The saturation level of concern has been defined as <30% based on animal and human data. Acidosis tends to set in only if the value is <30% for a period of more than 10 min.[158]

The first randomized study, using the algorithm shown in Table 13.3, consisted of 1010 women. It showed a reduction in operative delivery for fetal distress but there was no reduction in the overall caesarean section rate.[152] This trial established that an oxygen saturation of >30% was associated with a fetus without metabolic acidosis. A new sensor, with a scalp electrode, has been developed and it is expected to increase the percentage of continuous recordings in labour. However a recent large randomized study of 5341 nulliparous women did not show any difference in caesarean section rate or of the neonatal condition between groups.[159] Of greater interest in this study was that 34.6% of cases with non-reassuring traces and 25.1%

Table 13.3 Algorithm for using cardiotocography (CTG) and peripheral saturation of oxygen (SpO$_2$) in labour

CTG	Fetal SpO$_2$	Action	Comments
Normal	—	Continue labour	No need for SpO$_2$
Severe bradycardia	—	Deliver for fetal distress	Do not wait for SpO$_2$
Non-reassuring	>30%	Continue labour	Fetus is adequately oxygenated Consider corrective measures
Non-reassuring	<30%	Observe for 10 min	Apply corrective measures Change maternal position Correct hypotension Reduce oxytocic drugs Consider tocolytics/O$_2$
Non-reassuring	<30% for 10 min	Apply corrective measures If no improvement deliver	May use fetal scalp pH to confirm fetal status

of cases with normal reassuring traces had low oxygen saturation, defined as an oxygen saturation <30% for longer than 2 min. The lack of benefit, of not reducing the caesarean section rate, without any improvement in the neonatal outcome, based on two randomized studies casts doubt about the efficacy and use of pulse oximetry in labour.

DOPPLER ULTRASOUND

The benefit of Doppler umbilical artery blood flow recording as a tool for antenatal assessment of fetal wellbeing in high risk pregnancies has been documented in several studies.[160,161] A semiquantitative blood flow class system, describing blood velocity waveform with emphasis on the end-diastolic part, was the most powerful marker of imminent fetal asphyxia and of intrauterine growth restriction. In experimental asphyxia in fetal lambs, aortic mean blood flow velocities were reduced. Aortic blood flow waveforms showed low end-diastolic flow velocities and/or increased pulsatility indices (PI).[162] In the common carotid artery of the fetuses, the PI tended to decrease during asphyxia and the umbilical artery PI remained unchanged. The changes in the fetal aortic velocity waveforms indicate an adaptation of the peripheral circulation to asphyxia. The waveform changes seem to be a late phenomenon in the process of asphyxia.

Doppler ultrasound of the umbilical artery flow velocity waveform was studied prospectively as an admission test at the labour ward in 575 women in various stages of labour before, during and after uterine contractions, and evaluated in relation to intrapartum and fetal outcome variables.[62] Fetuses who are small for gestational age had significantly more abnormal blood flow velocity waveforms than did fetuses who were appropriate for gestational age, and more patients with umbilical artery acidemia had abnormal blood flow velocity waveforms compared with those with normal pH. However, no association was found between abnormal flow velocity waveforms and cord complications, meconium-stained amniotic fluid or abnormal FHR tracing; nor was there any association with operative delivery for fetal distress or low Apgar scores at 1 min and 5 min. Doppler recording of the umbilical artery flow velocity waveform as an admission test at the labour ward was not a good predictor of fetal distress.

A patient with a small-for-gestational-age fetus at 36 weeks had a non-stress test (NST) that showed a non-reactive trace. However, the umbilical artery Doppler velocity waveform showed normal blood flow (Fig. 13.7). Because of the clinical picture (fundosymphysis height of 30 cm at 36 weeks and clinically reduced amniotic fluid) and a non-reactive NST, labour was induced. The cervix was 1 cm long and 1 cm dilated. On rupture of the membranes there was scanty but clear amniotic fluid. With 2.5 mU/min of oxytocin, contractions of 1 in 2–3 min occurred and with each contraction there were variable to late decelerations (Fig. 13.8). The baby was delivered by caesarean section, weighed 1.8 kg and had an Apgar score of 9 at both 1 and 5 min and a cord arterial pH of 7.28. Although the baby was in good condition, with the given clinical picture and the FHR tracing it would have been unwise to continue labour, although the Doppler velocity waveform was reassuring.

Doppler blood flow measurements in labour appear to be useful in evaluating the effects of drugs on uterine and fetal blood flow, but have little to contribute to routine intrapartum fetal monitoring. Sophisticated equipment, as well as trained personnel, are needed to perform good measurements, making this method difficult to implement in a continuous form or even as an intermittent method in labour.

CONTINUOUS pH MEASUREMENTS

Much effort has been expended over many years to develop a continuous pH electrode and to perform continuous pH measurements in labour. This has been fraught with technical difficulties. The electrodes tend to be large, difficult to apply and fragile. Furthermore,

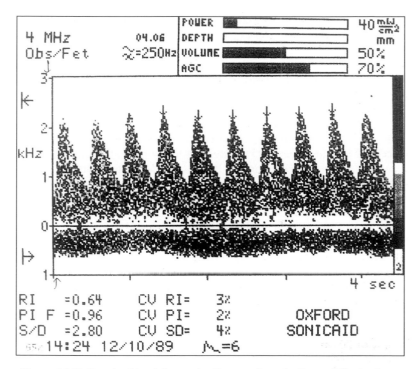

Figure 13.7 Doppler blood flow velocity waveform in the umbilical artery of a growth-restricted fetus at term

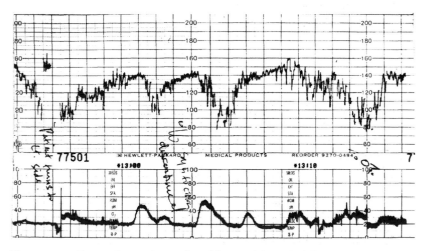

Figure 13.8 Trace of growth-restricted fetus with normal Doppler results showing variable and late decelerations with commencement of oxytocin for induction of labour

there appears to be a drift in the value when the electrode is in place over a long period of time. Caput formation and venous stasis can affect the readings. It is not uncommon to find occasional low pH of a respiratory type in a healthy baby during labour which tends to recover on its own with passage of time. In studies dealing with pH in labour the mean pH is calculated from a large number of fetuses. The mean acid–base values from 130 cases of low-risk labour are given in Table 13.4.[163]

In this series there were individual cases with low pH values (Table 13.5), but since the FHR recordings were satisfactory labour was allowed to progress and the babies were delivered vaginally. At delivery the Apgar scores were good and the cord pH values were not acidotic, indicating that transient changes in pH are not an

Table 13.4 Acid-base values in scalp and cord blood (mean value)

	Cervical dilatation		Cord arterial blood
	5 cm	10 cm	
pH	7.332	7.335	7.292
PCO_2	66.85	66.87	50.56
PO_2	25.00	24.06	21.05
HCO_3	24.15	23.93	23.08

HCO_3, bicarbonate; PCO_2, partial pressure of carbon dioxide; PO_2, partial pressure of oxygen

Table 13.5 Distribution of pH values in scalp and cord blood

	Cervical dilatation				Cord arterial blood	
	5 cm		10 cm			
pH	n	%	n	%	n	%
<7.10	–	–	–	–	2	1.7
<7.15	1	0.8	2	1.7	4	3.4
<7.20	2	1.7	3	2.5	9	7.5
<7.25	7	5.8	7	5.8	31	25.8
<7.30	31	25.8	28	23.7	61	50.8
>7.30	89	74.8	90	76.3	59	49.2

uncommon finding in any labour: these changes are mostly of a respiratory type and will correct themselves with time. From a large series in the UK[120] it was reported that 73% of infants with cord arterial pH below 7.10 had a 1-min Apgar score of over 7, and 86% had a 5-min Apgar score over 7. Low arterial pH is usually due to accumulation of carbon dioxide and its influence on pH. Respiratory acidosis is poorly correlated with fetal or neonatal condition. Clearly, it would be difficult to manage patients on continuous pH measurements alone, and additional information on the blood gases is required. Information from the FHR pattern along with continuous pH measurements is unlikely to improve the present standards of intrapartum fetal surveillance, unless base excess values are known in order to define whether it is respiratory or metabolic acidosis, as there is a significant drop and quick recovery of pH due to respiratory acidosis.

LACTATE

Measurement of lactate needed large volumes of blood in the past. With advances in technology and sports medicine, measurement of lactate using 5 µl of blood has become a reality. Lactate is produced within the cell when there is lack of oxygen and there is anaerobic metabolism. This takes a long time to develop and takes much longer to eliminate as it has to be cleared through the placenta.[164] Since this is a true marker of metabolic acidosis, trials are in progress to establish this method in intrapartum surveillance.

There are different types of equipment available for measuring lactate and the normal ranges of scalp and cord blood lactate vary slightly with each machine.[165] The one with which a lot of work has been done is the 'Lactate Pro' equipment and a level of >4.8 mmol/L is considered abnormal with this equipment.[166] Compared with 35 µl needed for pH and base excess measurement, these machines require only 5 µl. Trials have shown that blood collection for lactate is more successful, needs less scalp incisions and is much quicker to get the result by the bedside.[167]

Studies conducted in Sweden correlated cord arterial lactate measurements to immediate and long-term outcome of neonates (two-year follow up) and have shown it to be a reliable surrogate marker of neonatal outcome.[168] One randomized controlled trial compared scalp blood pH versus lactate, which showed less failure rates and less babies with severe metabolic acidosis in the lactate group.[167] Further large randomized studies in other centres are needed to establish whether the same results can be reproduced. The results of such studies are not forthcoming and may be an indication of the reluctance of the caregivers and the mothers to accept an invasive procedure of fetal scalp blood sampling.

STIMULATION TESTS

Fetal acoustic and scalp stimulation tests have been used as adjunctive forms of testing with the CTG in intrapartum surveillance. This has been discussed in detail in Chapter 12.

Any new method of fetal surveillance generates great enthusiasm when first applied. Caution must be exercised before wider clinical implementation. It should be recognized that new methods may involve greater invasion and inconvenience for the woman and should not be used unless the person is trained adequately and has a good knowledge of the technology.

Chapter 14

Computer technology and the cardiotocograph

Computers have become a central part of modern life. In pregnancy care their value lies in display, transmission, storage and, to a lesser extent, analysis of data. They have a clear educational role, potentially using the limitless possibilities of internet technology.

Sophisticated viewing systems allow the display of data at a central delivery suite location. This allows overviewing of all monitors in the unit and selective display of further information on any particular monitor. The advantage of this is that it allows further opinion or concern to be voiced about any particular trace by a supervisor or another third party. In analysis of mistakes made in cardiotocograph (CTG) interpretation, human error of one person involved has been recognized. One person on the day may have personal stresses, be feeling below par or have other reason to perform suboptimally. Support is important. The disadvantage of this central system is that it may cause managers to downgrade the priority for one-to-one care. The place of the midwife is beside the bed: the central monitor should not remove the need for the bedside midwife. The midwife has so many other important roles apart from watching the monitor.

These displays incorporate alert and alarm signals which can be set at particular levels locally. However, experience shows that the variety of intrapartum fetal heart rate (FHR) patterns seen and clinical scenarios experienced do not facilitate the use of such a framework. It is common for midwives and doctors to use such devices initially but later to turn them off or, worse, ignore them. Remember the mother and her partner are watching what is happening. More and more they are asking about the CTG and what it is showing. Ignoring apparent alerts does not inspire confidence.

Failure to document events in labour is common. It is important to document the date and time of each event in labour and the interrelationship of the FHR pattern to vaginal examination findings, administration of drugs and other episodes. To facilitate this, the manufacturers of fetal monitors have produced equipment that self-annotates the FHR trace with the date, time and mode of recording (e.g. ultrasound, fetal electrocardiograph, external or internal toco-graph). A keypad or a bar-coded entry system can be attached to the fetal monitor to enable additional findings such as results of a vaginal examination, colour of amniotic fluid, etc. to be entered on the trace. The blood pressure and oxygen saturation can be entered automatically from the blood pressure monitor. Not only are the entered data printed on the trace but they are registered in the mother's obstetric notes which are maintained in the computer (with date and time of entry). This can be reviewed from time to time, updated or printed to obtain a hard copy. Based on the cervical examination findings entered by the bedside via the keypad of the fetal monitor, a partogram may be automatically drawn on the computer screen. These obstetric management systems not only keep the most wanted records but will also form a reserve for future research and to generate statistics. Most systems can keep up to 8 h of labour record notes and the FHR tracings of 4000 subjects in a small optical disc which can be kept for many years. Tampering with the records on a subsequent occasion is impossible. Though a costly investment, in the long run it will pay for itself even if it helps to solve only one medico-legal case in which the records have been lost using traditional methods of record keeping.

The distant transmission of a CTG over a telephone system may be appropriate in some areas where distances are great, and can be a way to obtain a second opinion. This can also be achieved by a fax transmission of the CTG. This should not be used as a reason to do more CTGs on normal pregnancies: it may however provide a rapid channel to a second opinion of a more senior person. Using the Internet to transmit this information will open up greater possibilities.

Computers offer limitless possibilities for storage, archiving and retrieval of data. Obstetric records are now generally computerized after years of development. Unfortunately midwives often find that time spent at the computer is just more paperwork and time spent away from the mother and her baby. This is another challenge. Although not yet commonly linked with the obstetric record, the electronic storage of the CTG is feasible. This is certainly done in the antenatal scenario with the use of devices like the Oxford Sonicaid System 8000. The most important reason to store and be able to retrieve the CTG effectively is the possibility of litigation in cases with an adverse outcome. A hard copy original CTG fades in a few years depending on the storage environment. After an adverse incident an immediate photocopy should be made of the continuous CTG. The photocopy does not fade!

Can computers assist in analysis and decision making? Data may be processed to provide indices of the FHR other than those previously discussed. The Oxford Sonicaid System 8000 performs this function on antenatal FHR recordings. It provides a screen display of the CTG and also stores every trace recorded on a hard drive. This information can be recalled at short notice and provides a valuable system for research studies. The analysis system programmed by Dawes and Redman assesses various features of the tracing, defining accelerations as a rise in baseline of 10 beats for 10 s and assessing baseline variability as mean range.[169] Mean range of variation is considered the most important index: if it is greater than 20 ms it is normal. The information produced is highlighted as 'advisory only' and clinical decisions remain the responsibility of the clinician. Such programmes may have some value educationally and for research purposes; however, there is a danger they may be seen as a short cut to interpreting the CTG without proper understanding. The further danger is that staff will lose their skills in intrapartum CTG interpretation which cannot be subjected to the same computerized analysis. A comparison was made between the value, given as a score between 1 and 100, by an experienced observer for a series of antenatal CTGs and the Dawes Redman score. There was a high degree of agreement and a very strong correlation.[170]

Attempts have been made to devise a computer system to aid the interpretation of intrapartum CTGs. The problem has been the great variability in patterns of FHR depending on both physiological and pathological mechanisms. In addition the CTG cannot be separated from the clinical scenario. A multicentre study was performed comparing the opinion of 17 experts with the analysis of an intelligent computer system for managing labour using the CTG.[171] The system's performance was found to be indistinguishable from the experts' in the 50 cases examined, but it was more consistent. This demonstrates the potential for an intelligent computer system to improve the interpretation of the CTG and decrease intervention. Furthermore, the good performance of most experts in this study demonstrates the potential effectiveness of the CTG and raises important questions regarding why the CTG has fallen short of expectations in current practice.

The best analysis computer is the one most freely available in all labour wards: the human brain. It must be continuously optimized by education and training. This, in turn, can be aided by computers. More and more hospitals are implementing computerized training packages for staff. The use and proven completion of such a system can be linked to the continuing education certification of a midwife or doctor. More such packages and online education may become available in the future.

Chapter 15

Medico-legal issues

In the late 1980s few hospitals had guidelines of practice for obstetrics and midwifery. Now they are almost universal. Only to a small degree has this been due to an increasing evidence base for practice. To a greater degree it has been because of a desire to promote a better quality of care and counter what has been a rising tide of litigation. Safe childbirth is seen in modern society as a right. This has become an expectation. When it goes wrong people ask why this should happen to them. If they do not get a satisfactory answer from the hospital they turn to the law. We should try to understand why families take legal action and the nature of this action. It most often relates to a damaged child. Although financial support is part of the objective, every family would rather have a healthy child. The legal process itself is long and tedious. The family would much rather devote the precious time to looking after the injured child. The families often feel that they have not been given an explanation of what happened and communication has been poor. They also feel that what has happened to them should not happen to other people. We are sometimes asked if we practise defensive medicine. The answer is that good medicine is defensive medicine. If we practise according to guidelines with good communication and giving parents choices then this is the defence against litigation.

In the face of a huge tide of litigation, the National Health Service (NHS) turned its attention to this issue with the formation of the National Health Service Litigation Authority (NHSLA) as a special health authority in 1995. The NHSLA has four principal functions:

1. To ensure claims are dealt with consistently and with due regard to the proper interests of the NHS and its patients.
2. To manage the financial consequences of such claims.
3. To advise the Department of Health on both specific and general issues arising out of claims against the NHS.

4. To manage and raise the standards of risk management throughout the NHS.

In its current annual report the NHSLA state that despite widespread concerns about a 'compensation culture' in the UK, claims remain very steady with a 1.6% increase in clinical claims in 2005/2006.[172] These are overall claims. Obstetric claims remain the second largest group (after surgery) and the highest value. There is limited information about trends in obstetric claims. Of the clinical claims made against the NHS in the 10 years of the existence of the NHSLA, 43% of claims were settled out of court, 38% were abandoned by the claimant, 15% have yet to settle and 4% were settled in court. Fewer than 50 negligence cases a year are settled in court. Of the 87 clinical negligence cases actually litigated in court in the last two financial years, 26% were settled in court in favour of the claimant, 68% were settled in favour of the NHS and 6% settled mid trial.

The NHSLA take a very active role in risk management. The Clinical Negligence Scheme for Trusts (CNST) run by the NHSLA sets standards, most recently stated in the 'Maternity Clinical Risk Management Standards'.[173] These are endorsed both by the Royal College of Obstetricians and Gynaecologists and the Royal College of Midwives. These standards cover staffing levels and competence, clinical standards, administrative standards and reporting. Education, referral relationships, training and labour ward cover, including certified attendance at cardiotocograph educational meetings, are included. Achievement of these standards at an inspection, at intervals of 1, 2 and 3 years, is scored with a final attainment of a level 0, 1, 2 or 3. Trusts receive the financial incentive of a 10%, 20% or 30% reduction in their payments in future years into the scheme as a reward for higher level attainment. Currently 50% of trusts in England are at level 1, with 45% at level 2 and only about 5% at level 3 (the highest level). The bureaucracy of this consumes considerable time, money and effort which is sometimes diverted from clinical care.

When things go wrong there should be a local system of identification and support. Critical incident reporting has now become well established. The advantage of this is that reports are written very soon after the event and are more valid. Of course, case notes should contain the relevant details written contemporaneously. Staff can feel oppressed by the burden of reviewing any incident, however small, and the member of staff responsible for risk management locally should provide advice about this. An open and frank atmosphere should be encouraged. The NHSLA encourages apologies and explanations when things go wrong. This is crucial. Patients may be satisfied by a responsive and sympathetic complaints process. If they feel that they have not been listened to or have been treated unfairly then they may proceed to the litigation process.

There is a growing realism by hospital trusts that a move towards resolution sooner rather than later benefits everyone. This has also been recognized by the report to the Lord Chancellor by Lord Woolf (Lord Justice, Master of the Rolls) entitled *Access to Justice*.[174] Families should not suffer the stress of waiting for up to 10 years while the case goes through the system. Woolf criticized the cost, delays and confrontational attitude of opposing lawyers.

The legal process involves the establishing of liability, causation and quantum. So far as damage to a child is concerned, the time lapse before the commencement of litigation is unlimited. The child's claim is made by the mother, father or another adult on behalf of the child. Legally this person is called the child's 'next friend'. If the claim relates to damage to the mother then a limitation of 3 years applies. The mother (and any other party present) makes a statement as to what she believes happened or did not happen related to the damage which she alleges. A solicitor then conducts the legal process. The Law Society has established a panel of solicitors' firms with the expertise to undertake this work efficiently. Similarly the NHSLA has a panel of firms who have a similar expertise in the area allowing them to act effectively and efficiently for the defence. The clinical notes are requested from the hospital. These will be (have to be) exactly as compiled by the staff at the time. The importance of careful, legible note keeping is obvious. Regrettably, in many hospitals the standard is poor. Midwives in general keep very good notes. Junior doctors more often than not have illegible signatures and do not date and time their entry to the notes. At every interaction between a doctor and the mother an entry must be made. This should preferably be by the doctor involved.

A high standard of note keeping reflects a high standard of care.

When the records have been obtained from the hospital they are photocopied and the solicitor then instructs independent medical experts to consider the information. In the common instance of a handicapped child after childbirth, several experts require to be instructed. Midwifery, obstetric and neonatology experts may be required to consider liability. A report is prepared concerning the standard of care provided. This is currently measured according to the Bolam principle. Essentially this involves a view as to whether the practice adopted would be that adopted by a responsible body of medical opinion. This allows for the fact of the art as well as the science of medicine. There may be several ways of approaching the problem, but what has to be shown for a defence is that the approach adopted would be adopted by a significant number of other reasonable people. As guidelines become more and more established these will be the local standards. They are generally consistent with wider national or international standards. The importance of orientation of new, and temporary, staff and their familiarity with the guidelines is obvious. This forms part of the CNST standards.

Paediatric neurology and imaging experts will be required for the determination of causation. This essentially considers whether the alleged result, the condition today, of the child can be considered on the balance of probability to be due to the alleged event for which the staff are liable. There are many natural factors that may result in damage to a child. The most frequent one is prematurity. In many cases this appears to have been unavoidable irrespective of the standard of care. In congenital abnormality associated with handicap, poor management of labour or misinterpretation of the cardiotocograph may have made little difference to the outcome. A case that is strong on liability may fail on causation. Other experts are occasionally required when a related field of expertise is relevant (anaesthesia, for instance). Quantum is considered at a later stage to determine what facilities and support are required as a result of the injury and a full panoply of quantum experts may be required.

After the initial reports the instructing solicitor will call a case conference led by a barrister to consider whether the case merits further process. This has to be justified to the Legal Services Commission who only authorize expenses warranted by the case as presented by the barrister. This conference may result in the barrister drafting a Letter of Claim. A proportion will be discontinued after expert opinion has recommended that there is no case to pursue. During this time the defendant hospital should have identified a possible claim and obtained statements and independent expert opinion of their own. A proportion will be settled by the defending hospital trust with a recognition that the case will be difficult to defend in court. Early resolution limits costs. Mediation or formal negotiations may be appropriate at any stage of the process. The defence solicitors will provide a Letter of Response to the Letter of Claim. This will cover the matters agreed and the matters not agreed with reasons. These letters will be further discussed by the claimants' legal advisors and a decision made about whether to issue formal legal proceedings with a claim form issued at court. Particulars of Claim will be formalized based on the original Letter of Claim. The defence team will respond with a defence. At this stage there will be an exchange of witness statements followed by an exchange of expert witness evidence. Since the Woolf reforms there is the additional opportunity for a meeting of experts to try to narrow the issues down. After that there is a round table meeting of the opposing legal teams to try to reach a final settlement and avoid court proceedings. It can be seen that every effort is made to avoid costly and emotionally traumatic court proceedings.

The above system applies only to England. In Scotland expert evidence is not exchanged prior to trial and there is less opportunity for resolution before appearing at court. There are also important differences in other countries. Since the Woolf reforms there have been important improvements in the system. An area that still requires reform is the system of expert witnesses. There is no question that such experts are required in the present system. They must be fair and unbiased. They should not act as an advocate for one side or the other: they are there to assist the court. They are obliged to sign a declaration and can be exposed to public reprimand by the judge if they do not fulfil their role properly. One problem is that experts are retained by one side or the other and, just as there are solicitors' firms that act for only one side or the other, so do they have contacts in experts who do the same. Experts have not been regulated, although there are at least two professional bodies to which they subscribe: The Expert Witness Institute and The Academy of Experts. There is an increasing structure of training and accreditation for experts. It is important that new experts enter this rewarding and interesting field.

People have to be incentivised in risk management. Too often the bureaucracy becomes unwieldy with ever more regulation. There are several national organisations interested in patient safety. The result is that there has now had to be a voluntary agreement to coordinate the various regulatory bodies: the concordat between bodies inspecting, regulating and auditing health care.

Litigation can be reduced by good standards of care and good communication. Surely this is something to which we should aspire even without a legal threat.

Chapter 16

Conclusion

After fifteen years, three editions of this book and uncountable teaching sessions and seminars our philosophy is essentially unchanged.

There is little doubt that electronic fetal heart rate (FHR) monitoring is likely to stay because of the uncertainties of the other methods due to technical difficulties and the limited correlation of the results obtained to the clinical outcome. Contraction monitoring is likely to be by external tocography in the majority of cases. Until a perfect method is developed to identify intrapartum hypoxia, we should learn to correlate the FHR pattern with the clinical picture in order to plan the management for each individual case. More time should be devoted to educate ourselves in FHR trace interpretation because our daily practice requires this. Failure to do so may lead to unnecessary caesarean sections or results in babies with birth asphyxia due to misinterpretation of the FHR trace. The benefits of intrapartum fetal monitoring in the future depend on formal education in trace interpretation, which has been sadly lacking. This should be in parallel to research in pursuit of better methods of fetal surveillance.

Cardiotocography is useful if:

- adequate knowledge is available to interpret the trace
- its limitations are known
- it is used appropriately
- the clinical picture is incorporated
- additional tests are used when in doubt
- common sense prevails.

We must not let technology dehumanize us: we must humanize technology.

STOP PRESS: further information about classification of fetal heart rate features

As the book went to press, NICE Clinical Guideline 55 was issued: see Table 4.1 on p. 43 for details. The following further information about classifying fetal heart rate traces is based on this Guideline:

- If repeated accelerations are present with reduced variability, the FHR trace should be regarded as reassuring.
- True early uniform decelerations are rare and benign, and therefore they are not significant.
- Most decelerations in labour are variable.
- If a bradycardia occurs in the baby for more than 3 min, urgent medical aid should be sought and preparations should be made to urgently expedite the birth of the baby, classified as a category 1 birth. This could include moving the woman to theatre if the fetal heart has not recovered by 9 min. If the fetal heart recovers within 9 min, the decision to deliver should be reconsidered in conjunction with the woman, if reasonable.
- A tachycardia in the baby of 160–180 bpm, where accelerations are present and no other adverse features appear, should not be regarded as suspicious; however, an increase in the baseline heart rate, even within the normal range, with other non-reassuring or abnormal features should increase concern.

References

1. Maternal and Child Health Research Consortium (MCHRC). Confidential enquiry into stillbirths and deaths in infancy. 4th annual report. London: MCHRC; 1997.
2. Macdonald D, Grant A, Sheridan-Perelra M, et al. The Dublin randomised controlled trial of intrapartum fetal heart rate monitoring. Am J Obstet Gynecol 1985; 152:524–539.
3. Leveno KJ, Cunningham FG, Nelson S, et al. A prospective comparison of selective and universal electronic fetal monitoring in 34995 pregnancies. N Engl J Med 1986; 315:615–619.
4. Department of Health. Changing childbirth. London: HMSO; 1993.
5. Confidential Enquiry into Maternal and Child Health. Why mothers die 2000–2002. The sixth report of the confidential enquiries into maternal deaths in the United Kingdom. London: RCOG Press.
6. Belizan JM, Vittar J, Nardin JC, et al. Diagnosis of intrauterine growth retardation by a simple clinical method: measurement of uterine height. Am J Obstet Gynecol 1978; 131:643–646.
7. Bennet MJ. Antenatal fetal monitoring. In: Chamberlain GVP, ed. Contemporary obstetrics and gynaecology. London: Northwood Publications; 1977:117–124.
8. Boddy K, Parboosingh IJT, Shepherd WC. A schematic approach to antenatal care. Edinburgh: Edinburgh University; 1976.
9. Calvert PJ, Crean EE, Newcombe RG, et al. Antenatal screening by measurement of symphysis-fundus height. Br Med J (Clin Res Ed) 1982; 285:846–849.
10. Tikkanen M, Nuutila M, Hiilesmaa V, et al. Clinical presentation and risk factors of placental abruption. Acta Obstet Gynecol Scand 2006; 85:700–705.
11. Sherman DJ, Frenkel E, Kurzweil Y, et al. Characteristics of maternal heart rate patterns during labor and delivery. Obstet Gynecol 2002; 99:542–547.
12. International Federation of Obstetrics and Gynaecology (FIGO). Guidelines for the use of fetal monitoring. Int J Gynecol Obstet 1987; 25:159–167.
13. National Institute for Health and Clinical Excellence (NICE). The use of electronic fetal monitoring: the use and interpretation of cardiotocography in intrapartum fetal surveillance. NICE inherited clinical guideline C.

London: NICE; 2001. Online. Available: http://guidance.nice.org.uk/ CGC/niceguidance/html. Accessed March 2007.

14. Parer JT. In defense of FHR monitoring's specificity. Cont Obstet Gynaecol 1982; 19:228–234.

15. Fleischer A, Schulman H, Jagani N, et al. The development of fetal acidosis in the presence of an abnormal fetal heart rate tracing. I. The average for gestation age fetus. Am J Obstet Gynecol 1982; 144:55–60.

16. Wheeler T, Murills A. Patterns of fetal heart rate during normal pregnancy. Br J Obstet Gynaecol 1978; 85:18–27.

17. Spencer JAD, Johnson P. Fetal heart rate variability changes and fetal behavioural cycles during labour. Br J Obstet Gynaecol 1986; 93:314–321.

18. Schifrin B, Artenos J, Lyseight N. Late-onset fetal cardiac decelerations associated with fetal breathing movements. J Matern Fetal Neonatal Med 2002; 12(4):253–259.

19. Gardosi J. Customised growth charts. Gestation Network. Online. Available: http://www.gestation.net. Accessed March 2007.

20. Grant A, Elbourne D, Valentin L, et al. Routine formal fetal movement counting and risk of antepartum late death in normally formed singletons. Lancet 1989; 2(8659):345–349.

21. Sadovsky E, Yaffe H, Polishuk WZ. Fetal movements in pregnancy and urinary oestriol in prediction of impending fetal death in utero. Isr J Med Sci 1974; 10:1096–1099.

22. Sadovsky E, Yaffe H. Daily fetal movement recordings and fetal prognosis. Obstet Gynecol 1973; 41:845–850.

23. Sadovsky E. Monitoring fetal movements: a useful screening test. Cont Obstet Gynaecol 1985; 25:123–127.

24. Sadovsky E, Rabinowitz R, Yaffe H. Decreased foetal movements and foetal malformations. J Foetal Med 1981; 1:62–64.

25. Fong YS, Kuldip S, Malcus P, et al. Assessment of fetal health should be based on maternal perception of clusters rather than episodes of fetal movements. J Obstet Gynaecol Res 1996; 22:299–304.

26. Stanco LM, Rabello Y, Medearis AL, et al. Does Doppler-detected fetal movement decrease the incidence of nonreactive nonstress tests? Obstet Gynecol 1993; 82:999–1003.

27. Patrick J, Carmichael L, Laurie C, et al. Accelerations of the human fetal heart rate at 38 to 40 weeks' gestational age. Am J Obstet Gynecol 1984; 148:35–41.

28. Kubli F, Boos R, Ruttgers H, et al. Antepartum fetal heart rate monitoring and ultrasound in obstetrics. In: Beard RW, ed. Royal College of Obstetricians and Gynaecologists (RCOG) Scientific Meeting. London: RCOG; 1977:28–47.

29. Schifrin BS, Foye G, Amato J, et al. Routine fetal heart rate monitoring in the antepartum period. Obstet Gynecol 1979; 54:21–25.

30. Keagan KA, Paul RH. Antepartum fetal heart rate monitoring: non-stress test as a primary approach. Am J Obstet Gynecol 1980; 136:75–80.

31. Flynn AM, Kelly J, Mansfield H, et al. A randomised controlled trial of non-stress antepartum cardiotocography. Br J Obstet Gynaecol 1982; 89:427–433.

32. Smith CB, Phelan JP, Paul RH, et al. Fetal acoustic stimulation testing: a retrospective experience with the fetal acoustic stimulation test. Am J Obstet Gynecol 1985; 153:567–568.

33. Smith CV, Phelan JP, Platt LD, et al. Acoustic stimulation testing II. A randomized clinial comparison with the non-stress test. Am J Obstet Gynecol 1986; 155:131–134.
34. Schiff E, Lipitz S, Sivan E, et al. Acoustic stimulation as a diagnostic test: comparison with oxytocin challenge test. J Perinat Med 1992; 20:275–279.
35. Chamberlain PF, Manning FA, Morrison I, et al. Ultrasound evaluation of amniotic fluid (Vol. 1). The relationship of marginal and decreased amniotic fluid volumes to perinatal outcome. Am J Obstet Gynecol 1984; 150:245–249.
36. Crowley P, O'Herlihy C, Boylon P. The value of ultrasound measurement of amniotic fluid volume on the management of prolonged pregnancies. Br J Obstet Gynaecol 1984; 91:444–445.
37. Phelan JP, Ahn MO, Smith CV, et al. Amniotic fluid index measurements during pregnancy. J Reprod Med 1987; 32:601–604.
38. Jeng CJ, Jou TJ, Wang KG, et al. Amniotic fluid index measurements with the four quadrant technique during pregnancy. J Reprod Med 1990; 35:674–677.
39. Rutherford SE, Phelan JP, Smith CV, et al. The four quadrant assessment of amniotic fluid volume: an adjunct to antepartum fetal heart rate testing. Obstet Gynecol 1987; 70:353–356.
40. Moore TR, Cayle JE. The amniotic fluid index in normal human pregnancy. Am J Obstet Gynecol 1990; 162:1168–1173.
41. Moore TR. Superiority of the four quadrant sum over the single deepest pocket technique in ultrasonographic identification of abnormal amniotic fluid volumes. Am J Obstet Gynecol 1990; 163:762–767.
42. Rutherford SE, Smith CV, Phelan JP, et al. Four quadrant assessment of amniotic fluid volume. Inter-observer and intra-observer variation. J Reprod Med 1987; 32:587–589.
43. Clark SL, Sabey P, Jolly K. Nonstress testing with acoustic stimulation and amniotic fluid volume assessment: 5973 tests without unexpected fetal death. Am J Obstet Gynecol 1989; 160:694–697.
44. Anandakumar C, Biswas A, Arulkumaran S, et al. Should assessment of amniotic fluid volume form an integral part of antenatal fetal surveillance of high risk pregnancy? Aust N Z J Obstet Gynaecol 1993; 33:272–275.
45. Vintzileos AM, Fleming AD, Scorza WE, et al. Relationship between fetal biophysical activities and cord blood gas values. Am J Obstet Gynecol 1991; 165:707–712.
46. Manning FA, Platt LD, Sipos L. Antepartum fetal evaluation: development of a biophysical profile. Am J Obstet Gynecol 1980; 136:787–790.
47. Manning FA, Morrison I, Harman CR, et al. Fetal assessment based on fetal biophysical profile scoring: experience in 19 221 referred high risk pregnancies. Am J Obstet Gynecol 1987; 157:880–884.
48. Johnson JM, Hareman CR, Lange IR, et al. Biophysical scoring in the management of postterm pregnancy: an analysis of 307 patients. Am J Obstet Gynecol 1986; 154:269–273.
49. Eden RD, Seifert LS, Koack LD, et al. A modified biophysical profile for antenatal fetal surveillance. Obstet Gynecol 1988; 71:365–369.
50. Maeda K. Computerized analysis of cardiotocograms and fetal movements. Baillière's Clin Obstet Gynaecol 1990; 4:797–813.
51. Timor-Trisch IE, Dierker LJ, Zador RH, et al. Fetal movements associated with fetal heart rate accelerations. Am J Obstet Gynecol 1978; 131:276–281.

52. Montan S, Arulkumaran S, Ratnam SS. Evaluation of a simple method to assess fetal well-being in antenatal clinic. J Perinat Med 1994; 22:175–180.

53. Drew JH, Kelly E, Chew FTK, et al. Prospective study of the quality of survival of infants with critical reserve detected by antenatal cardiotocography. Aust N Z J Obstet Gynaecol 1992; 32:32–35.

54. Navot D, Mor-Yosef S, Granat M, et al. Antepartum fetal heart rate pattern associated with major congenital malformations. Obstet Gynecol 1983; 63:414–417.

55. Buchdahl R, Hird M, Gibb D, et al. Listeriosis revisited: the role of the obstetrician. Br J Obstet Gynaecol 1990; 97:186–189.

56. Hobel CJ, Hyvarinen MA, Okada DM, et al. Prenatal and intrapartum high risk screening. 1. Prediction of the high risk neonate. Am J Obstet Gynecol 1973; 117:1–9.

57. Arulkumaran S, Gibb DMF, Ratnam SS. Experience with a selective intrapartum fetal monitoring policy. Singapore J Obstet Gynecol 1983; 14:47–51.

58. Ingemarsson I, Arulkumaran S, Ingemarsson E, et al. Admission test: a screening test for fetal distress in labour. Obstet Gynecol 1986; 68:800–806.

59. Bix E, Reiner LM, Klovning A, et al. Prognostic value of the labour admission test and its effectiveness compared with auscultation only: a systematic review. Br J Obstet Gynaecol 2005; 112:1595–1604.

60. Mires G, Williams F, Howie P. Randomised controlled trial of cardiotocography versus Doppler auscultation of fetal heart at admission in labour in low risk obstetric population. BMJ 2001; 322:1435–1498.

61. Impey L, Reynolds M, MacQuillan K, et al. Admission cardiotocography: a randomised controlled trial. Lancet 2003; 361(9356):465–470.

62. Malcus P, Gudmundson S, Marsal K, et al. Umbilical artery Doppler velocimetry as a labour admission test. Obstet Gynecol 1991; 77:10–16.

63. Sarno APJ, Ahn MO, Brar H, et al. Intrapartum Doppler velocimetry, amniotic fluid volume and fetal heart rate as predictors of subsequent fetal distress. Am J Obstet Gynecol 1989; 161:1508–1511.

64. Chauchan SP, Washburne JF, Magann EF, et al. A randomized study to assess the efficacy of the amniotic fluid index as a fetal admission test. Obstet Gynecol 1995; 86:9–13.

65. Teoh TG, Gleeson RP, Darling MR. Measurement of amniotic fluid volume in early labour is a useful admission test. Br J Obstet Gynaecol 1992; 99:859–860.

66. Chua S, Arulkumaran S, Kurup A, et al. Search for the most predictive tests of fetal well-being in early labour. J Perinat Med 1996; 24:199–206.

67. Chan FY, Lam C, Lam YH, et al. Umbilical artery Doppler velocimetry compared with fetal heart rate monitoring as a labor admission test. Eur J Obstet Gynecol Reprod Biol 1994; 54:1–6.

68. Keegan KAJ, Waffarn F, Quilligan EJ. Obstetric characteristics and fetal heart rate patterns of infants who convulse during the newborn period. Am J Obstet Gynecol 1985; 153:732–737.

69. Van der Merwe P, Gerretsen G, Visser G. Fixed heart rate pattern after intrauterine accidental decerebration. Obstet Gynecol 1985; 65:125–127.

70. Menticoglou SM, Manning FA, Harman CR, et al. Severe fetal brain injury without evident intrapartum trauma. Obstet Gynecol 1989; 74:457–461.

71. Schields JR, Schifrin BS. Perinatal antecedents of cerebral palsy. Obstet Gynecol 1988; 71:899–905.
72. Leveno KJ, William ML, De Palma RT, et al. Perinatal outcome in the absence of antepartum fetal heart rate accelerations. Obstet Gynecol 1983; 61:347–355.
73. Devoe LD, McKenzie J, Searle NS, et al. Clinical sequelae of the extended non-stress test. Am J Obstet Gynecol 1985; 151:1074–1078.
74. Brown R, Patrick J. The non-stress test: how long is long enough? Am J Obstet Gynecol 1981; 141:646–651.
75. Phelan JP, Ahn MO. Perinatal observations in forty-eight neurologically impaired term infants. Am J Obstet Gynecol 1994; 171:424–431.
76. Herbst A, Ingemarsson I. Intermittent versus continuous electronic fetal monitoring in labour. Br J Obstet Gynaecol 1994; 101:663–668.
77. Arulkumaran S, Yeoh SC, Gibb DMF, et al. Obstetric outcome of meconium stained liquor in labour. Singapore Med J 1985; 26:523–526.
78. Steer PJ. Fetal distress. In: Crawford J, ed. Risks of labour. Chichester: John Wiley; 1985:11–31.
79. Hannah EM, Hannah WJ, Hewson SA, et al. Planned caesarean section versus planned vaginal birth for breech presentation at term: a randomised multicentre trial. Term Breech Trial Collaborative Group. Lancet 2000; 356(9239):1375–1383.
80. Montan S, Solum T, Sjoberg NO. Influence of the beta 1-adrenoceptor blocker atenolol on antenatal cardiotocography. Acta Obstet Gynecol Scand Suppl 1984; 118:99–102.
81. Melchior J, Bernard N. Second stage fetal heart rate patterns. In: Spencer JAD, ed. Fetal monitoring – physiology and techniques of antenatal and intrapartum assessment. Tunbridge Wells: Castle House Publications; 1989:155–158.
82. Bloom SL, Leveno KJ, Sponge CY, et al. Decision-to-incision times and maternal and infant outcomes. Obstet Gynecol 2006; 108:6–11.
83. Livermore LJ, Cochrane RM. Decision to delivery interval: A retrospective study of 1000 emergency caesarean sections. J Obstet Gynaecol 2006; 26(4):307–310.
84. Tuffnel JD, Wilkinson K, Beresford N. Interval between decision and delivery by caesarean section. BMJ 2001; 322:1330–1333.
85. MacKenzie IZ, Cooke I. What is reasonable time from decision to delivery be caesarean section? Evidence from 415 deliveries. Br J Obstet Gynaecol 2002; 109:498–504.
86. Royal College of Obstetricians and Gynaecologists (RCOG). The future role of the consultant. London: RCOG Press; 2006.
87. Arulkumaran S, Yang M, Chia YT, et al. Reliability of intrauterine pressure measurements. Obstet Gynecol 1991; 78:800–802.
88. Caldeyro-Barcia R, Sica-Blanco Y, Poseiro JJ, et al. A quantitative study of the action of synthetic oxytocin on the pregnant human uterus. J Pharmacol Exp Ther 1957; 121(1):18–31.
89. Hon EH, Paul RH. Quantitation of uterine activity. Obstet Gynecol 1973; 42:368–370.
90. Steer PJ. The measurement and control of uterine contractions. In: Beard RW, ed. The current status of fetal heart rate monitoring and ultrasound in obstetrics. London: Royal College of Obstetricians and Gynaecologists; 1977:48–68.

91. Gibb DMF. Measurement of uterine activity in labour – clinical aspects. Br J Obstet Gynaecol 1993; 110:28–31.

92. Arulkumaran S, Gibb DMF, Ratnam SS, et al. Total uterine activity in induced labour – an index of cervical and pelvic tissue resistance. Br J Obstet Gynaecol 1985; 92:693–697.

93. Arulkumaran S, Chua S, Chua TM, et al. Uterine activity in dysfunctional labour and target uterine activity to be aimed with oxytocin titration. Asia Oceania J Obstet Gynaecol 1991; 17:101–106.

94. Chua S, Kurup A, Arulkumaran S, et al. Augmentation of labor: does internal tocography produce better obstetric outcome than external tocography? Obstet Gynecol 1990; 76:164–167.

95. Beckley S, Gee H, Newton JR. Scar rupture in labour after previous lower segment caesarean section: the role of uterine activity measurement. Br J Obstet Gynaecol 1991; 98:265–269.

96. Arulkumaran S, Chua S, Ratnam SS. Symptoms and signs with scar rupture: value of uterine activity measurements. Aust N Z J Obstet Gynaecol 1992; 32:208–212.

97. Gibb DMF, Arulkumaran S. Assessment of uterine activity. In: Whittle M, ed. Clinics in obstetrics and gynaecology. London: Baillière Tindall; 1987:111–130.

98. National Institute for Health and Clinical Excellence (NICE). Induction of labour: Clinical guidelines. London: Royal College of Obstetricians and Gynaecologists; 2001. Online. Available: http://guidance.nice.org.uk/CGD/guidance/pdf/English. Accessed March 2007.

99. Arulkumaran S, Ingemarsson I. Appropriate technology in intrapartum fetal surveillance. In: Studd JWW, ed. Progress in obstetrics and gynaecology. Edinburgh: Churchill Livingstone; 1990:127–140.

100. Ingemarsson I, Arulkumaran S, Ratnam SS. Single injection of terbutaline in term labor. 1. Effect on fetal pH in cases with prolonged bradycardia. Am J Obstet Gynecol 1985; 153:859–865.

101. Ingemarsson I, Arulkumaran S, Ratnam SS. Single injection of terbutaline in term labor. 2. Effect on uterine activity. Am J Obstet Gynecol 1985; 153:865–869.

102. Sica BY, Sala NL. Oxytocin. In: Caldeyro-Barcia R, Heller H, eds. Proceedings of an International Symposium London. Oxford: Pergamon Press; 1961:127–136.

103. Ferguson JKW. A study of the motility of the intact uterus at term. Surg Gynecol Obstet 1941; 73:359–366.

104. Arulkumaran S, Ratnam SS. Caesarean sections in the management of severe hypertensive disorders in pregnancy and eclampsia. Singapore J Obstet Gynecol 1988; 19:61–66.

105. Modanlou HD, Freeman RH. Sinusoidal fetal heart rate patterns; its definition and clinical significance. Am J Obstet Gynecol 1982; 142:1033–1038.

106. Arulkumaran S, Tham KF. Sinusoidal like fetal heart rate pattern – real time ultrasound may help in differential diagnosis. Acta Obstet Gynecol Scand 1988; 67:573.

107. Gray JH, Dumore DW, Luther ER. Sinusoidal fetal heart rate pattern associated with alphaprodine administration. Obstet Gynecol 1978; 52:678–679.

108. Arulkumaran S, Wong YC, Anandakumar C, et al. Sinusoidal like pattern associated with acute fetomaternal transfusion. Aust N Z J Obstet Gynaecol 1989; 29:364–365.

109. Boylan P. Sinusoidal-like tracing in fetus with rhesus hemolytic anemia. Am J Obstet Gynecol 1985; 145:892–893.

110. Murray ML. Maternal or fetal heart rate? Avoiding intrapartum misidentification. J Obstet Gynecol Neonatal Nurs 2004; 33:93–104.

111. Schiffrin BS. The CTG and the timing and mechanism of fetal neurological injuries. In: Arulkumaran S, Gardosi J, guest eds. Intrauterine surveillance of the fetus. Best Pract Res Clin Obstet Gynaecol 2004; 18(3):467–478.

112. Beard RW, Morris ED, Clayton SG. pH of fetal capillary blood as an indicator of the condition of the fetus. J Obstet Gynaecol Br Commonw 1967; 74:812–817.

113. Beard RW, Filshie GM, Knight CA, et al. The significance of the changes in the continuous fetal heart rate in the first stage of labour. J Obstet Gynaecol Br Commonw 1971; 78:865–881.

114. Ingemarsson E. Routine electronic fetal monitoring during labor. Acta Obstet Gynecol Scand 1981; 99:1–29.

115. Zalor RW, Quilligan EJ. The influence of scalp sampling on the caesarean section rate for fetal distress. Am J Obstet Gynecol 1979; 135:239–246.

116. Katz M, Mazor M, Insler V. Fetal heart rate patterns and scalp pH as predictors of fetal distress. Isr J Med Sci 1981; 17:260–265.

117. Paul RH, Suidan AK, Yeh SY, et al. Clinical fetal monitoring. VII. The evaluation and significance of intrapartum baseline variability. Am J Obstet Gynecol 1975; 123:206–210.

118. Schifrin BS, Dame L. Fetal heart rate patterns: prediction of Apgar score. JAMA 1972; 219:1322–1325.

119. Starks GC. Correlation of meconium stained amniotic fluid, early intrapartum fetal pH and Apgar scores as predictors of perinatal outcome. Obstet Gynecol 1980; 55:604–609.

120. Sykes GS, Molloy PM, Johnson P, et al. Do Apgar scores indicate asphyxia? Lancet 1982; 1(8270):494–496.

121. Nordstrom L, Arulkumaran S, Chua S, et al. Continuous maternal glucose infusion during labor: effects on maternal and fetal glucose and lactate levels. Am J Perinatol 1995; 12:357–362.

122. Huch A, Huch R, Rooth G. Guidelines for blood sampling and measurements of pH and blood gas values in obstetrics. Eur J Obstet Gynecol Reprod Biol 1994; 54:165–175.

123. Ingemarsson I, Ingemarsson E, Solum T, et al. Influence of occiput posterior position on the fetal heart rate pattern. Obstet Gynecol 1980; 55:301–306.

124. Clarke SL, Gimovsky ML, Miller FC. Fetal heart rate response to scalp blood sampling. Am J Obstet Gynecol 1983; 144:706–708.

125. Clarke SL, Gimovsky ML, Miller FC. The scalp stimulation test: a clinical alternative to fetal scalp blood sampling. Am J Obstet Gynecol 1984; 148:274–277.

126. Arulkumaran S, Ingemarsson I, Ratnam SS. Fetal heart rate response to scalp stimulation as a test for fetal wellbeing in labour. Asia Oceania J Obstet Gynaecol 1987; 13:131–135.

127. Edersheim TG, Hutson JM, Druzin ML, et al. Fetal heart rate response to vibratory acoustic stimulation predicts fetal pH in labor. Am J Obstet Gynecol 1987; 157:1557–1560.

128. Fisk NM, Nicolaidis P, Arulkumaran S, et al. Vibroacoustic stimulation is not associated with sudden fetal catecholamine release. Early Hum Dev 1991; 25:11–17.

129. Arulkumaran S, Skurr B, Tong H, et al. No evidence of hearing loss due to fetal acoustic stimulation test. Obstet Gynecol 1991; 78:283–285.

130. Spencer JAD, Deans A, Nicolaidis P, et al. Fetal response to vibroacoustic stimulation during low and high fetal heart rate variability episodes in late pregnancy. Am J Obstet Gynecol 1991; 165:86–90.

131. Clarke SL, Paul RH. Intrapartum fetal surveillance: the role of fetal scalp blood sampling. Am J Obstet Gynecol 1985; 153:717–720.

132. Ingemarsson I, Arulkumaran S. Reactive FHR response to sound stimulation in fetuses with low scalp blood pH. Br J Obstet Gynaecol 1989; 96:562–565.

133. Irion O, Stuckelberger P, Montquin JM, et al. Is intrapartum vibratory acoustic stimulation a valid alternative to fetal scalp pH determination. Br J Obstet Gynaecol 1996; 103:642–647.

134. Recommendations arising from the 26th Royal College of Obstetricians and Gynaecologists (RCOG) study group. In: Spencer JAD, ed. Intrapartum fetal surveillance. London: RCOG Press; 1993:387–393.

135. Dunphy BC, Robinson JN, Sheil OM, et al. Caesarean section for fetal distress, the interval from decision to delivery, and the relative risk of poor neonatal condition. Br J Obstet Gynaecol 1991; 11:241–244.

136. Gillmer MDG, Combe D. Intrapartum fetal monitoring practice in the United Kingdom. Br J Obstet Gynaecol 1979; 86:753–758.

137. Wheble AM, Gillmer MDG, Spencer JAD, et al. Changes in fetal monitoring practice in the UK: 1977–1984. Br J Obstet Gynaecol 1989; 96:1140–1147.

138. Westgate J, Greene KR. How well is fetal blood sampling used in clinical practice? Br J Obstet Gynaecol 1999; 106:774–782.

139. Rosen KG, Dagbjartsson A, Henriksson BA, et al. The relationship between circulating catecholamine and ST waveform in the fetal lamb electrocardiogram during hypoxia. Am J Obstet Gynecol 1984; 149:190–195.

140. Amer-Wahlin I, Yli B, Arulkumaran S. Foetal ECG and STAN technology – a review. Eur Clinics Obstet Gynaecol 2005; 1:61–73.

141. Lilja H, Arulkumaran S, Lindecrantz K, et al. Fetal ECG during labour; a presentation of a micro-processor based system. J Biomed Eng 1988; 10:348–350.

142. Arulkumaran S, Lilja H, Lindecrantz K, et al. Fetal ECG waveform analysis should improve fetal surveillance in labour. J Perinat Med 1990; 187:13–22.

143. MacLachlan NA, Harding K, Spencer JAD, et al. Fetal heart rate, fetal acidaemia and the T/QRS ratio of the fetal ECG in labour. Br J Obstet Gynaecol 1991; 99:26–31.

144. Westgate J, Harris M, Curnow JSH, et al. Randomised trial of cardiotocography alone or with ST waveform analysis for intrapartum monitoring. Lancet 1992; 340(8813):194–198.

145. Amer-Wahlin I, Hellsten C, Noren H, et al. Cardiotocography only versus ST analysis of fetal electrocardiogram for intrapartum monitoring: a Swedish randomised controlled trial. Lancet 2001; 358(9281):534–538.

146. Raymond SPW, Whitfield CR. Systolic time intervals of the fetal cardiac cycle. Baillière's Clin Obstet Gynaecol 1987; 1:185–201.
147. Hon EH, Koh KS. Electromechanical intervals of the fetal cardiac cycle. Clin Obstet Gynaecol 1979; 6:215–221.
148. Organ LW, Bernstein A, Smith KC, et al. The pre-ejection period of the fetal heart: patterns of change during labour. Am J Obstet Gynecol 1974; 120:49–55.
149. Hon EH, Murata Y, Zanini B, et al. Continuous microfilm display of the electromechanical intervals of the cardiac cycle. Obstet Gynecol 1974; 43:722–728.
150. Johnson N, Johnson VA, Fisher J, et al. Fetal monitoring with pulse oximetry. Br J Obstet Gynaecol 1991; 98:36–41.
151. Kuhnert M, Seelbach-Goebel B, Di Renzo GC, et al. Guidelines for the use of fetal pulse oximetry during labour and delivery. Prenat Neonatal Med 1998; 3:432–433.
152. Garite TJ, Dildy GA, McNamara H, et al. A multicenter controlled trial of fetal pulse oximetry in the intrapartum managment of nonreassuring fetal heart rate patterns. Am J Obstet Gynecol 2000; 183:1049–1058.
153. East CE, Dunster KR, Colditz PB, et al. Fetal oxygen saturation monitoring in labour: an analysis of 118 cases. Aust N Z J Obstet Gynaecol 1997; 37:397–401.
154. Chua S, Yam J, Razvi K, et al. Intrapartum fetal oxygen saturation monitoring in a busy labour ward. Eur J Obstet Gynecol Reprod Biol 1999; 82:185–189.
155. Yam J, Chua S, Arulkumaran S. Intrapartum fetal pulse oximetry. Part I. Principles and technical issues. Obstet Gynecol Surv 2000; 55:163–172.
156. Yam J, Chua S, Arulkumaran S. Intrapartum fetal pulse oximetry. Part II. Clinical applications. Obstet Gynecol Surv 2000; 55:173–183.
157. Chua S, Yeong SM, Razvi K, et al. Fetal oxygen saturation during labour. Br J Obstet Gynaecol 1997; 104:1080–1083.
158. Seelbach-Gobel B, Heupel M, Kuhnert M, et al. The prediction of fetal acidosis by means of intrapartum fetal oximetry. Am J Obstet Gynecol 1999; 180:73–81.
159. Bloom SL, Sponge CY, Thom E, et al. Fetal pulse oximetry and caesarean delivery. N Eng J Med 2006; 355:2195–2202.
160. Trudinger BJ, Giles WB, Cook CM. Flow velocity waveforms in the maternal uteroplacental and umbilical placental circulation. Am J Obstet Gynecol 1985; 152:155–163.
161. Laurin J, Marsal K, Persson PH, et al. Ultrasound measurements of fetal blood flow in predicting fetal outcome. Br J Obstet Gynaecol 1987; 94:940–948.
162. Malcus P, Hokegard KH, Kjellmer I, et al. The relationship between arterial blood velocity waveforms and acid–base status in the fetal lamb during experimental asphyxia. J Matern Fetal Investig 1991; 1:29–34.
163. Ingemarsson I, Arulkumaran S. Fetal acid base balance in low risk patients in labour. Am J Obstet Gynecol 1986; 155:66–69.
164. Nordstrom L, Arulkumaran S. Intrapartum fetal hypoxia and biochemical markers: a review. Obstet Gynecol Surv 1998; 53(10):645–657.
165. Yam J, Chua S, Razvi K, et al. Evaluation of a new portable system for cord lactate determination. Gynecol Obstet Invest 1998; 45:29–31.

166. Westgren M, Kublickas M, Kruger K. Role of lactate measurements during labour. Obstet Gynecol Surv 1998; 54(1):43–48.

167. Westgren M, Kruger K, Ek S, et al. Lactate compared with pH analysis at fetal scalp blood sampling: a prospective randomised study. Br J Obstet Gynaecol 1998; 105:29–33.

168. Kruger K, Hallberg B, Blennow M, et al. Predictive value of fetal scalp blood lactate concentration and pH as markers of neurological disability. Am J Obstet Gynecol 1999; 5:1072–1078.

169. Dawes GS, Redman CWG, Smith JH. Improvements in the registration and analysis of fetal heart records at the bedside. Br J Obstet Gynaecol 1985; 92:317–325.

170. Cheng LC, Gibb DMF, Ayaji R, et al. A comparison between computerised (mean range) and clinical visual cardiotocographic assessment. Br J Obstet Gynaecol 1992; 99:817–820.

171. Keith RDF, Beckley S, Garibaldi JM, et al. A multicentre comparative study of 17 experts and an intelligent computer system for managing labour using the cardiotocogram. Br J Obstet Gynaecol 1995; 102:688–700.

172. National Health Service Litigation Authority. Annual report. 2006. Online. Available: http://www.nhsla.com/Publications. Accessed March 2007.

173. National Health Service Litigation Authority. Clinical Negligence Scheme for Trusts. Maternity clinical risk management standards. 2006. Online. Available: http://www.nhsla.com/RiskManagement/CnstStandards. Accessed March 2007.

174. The Right Honourable the Lord Woolf, Master of the Rolls. Access to justice. Final report. 1996. Online. Available: http://www.dca.gov.uk/civil/final/index.htm. Accessed March 2007.

Index